SLEEP TO WIN

How Navy SEALs and Other High Performers Stay on Top

KIRK PARSLEY

Ordering Information: Quantity sales. Special discounts are available on multiple purchases by corporations, associations, and others.

For details, contact the "Special Sales Department" at the address above.

Sleep To Win, Kirk Parsley—1st edition, 2017

www.evolveglobalpublishing.com

Book Layout: © 2017 Evolve Global Publishing www.evolveglobalpublishing.com

ISBN: (Paperback)

ISBN: (Hardcover)

ISBN-13: (Createspace)

ISBN-10: (Createspace)

ISBN: (Smashwords)

ASIN: B071KBJRQ4 (Amazon Kindle)

This book is available on Barnes & Noble, Kobo, Apple iBooks (digital)

Contents

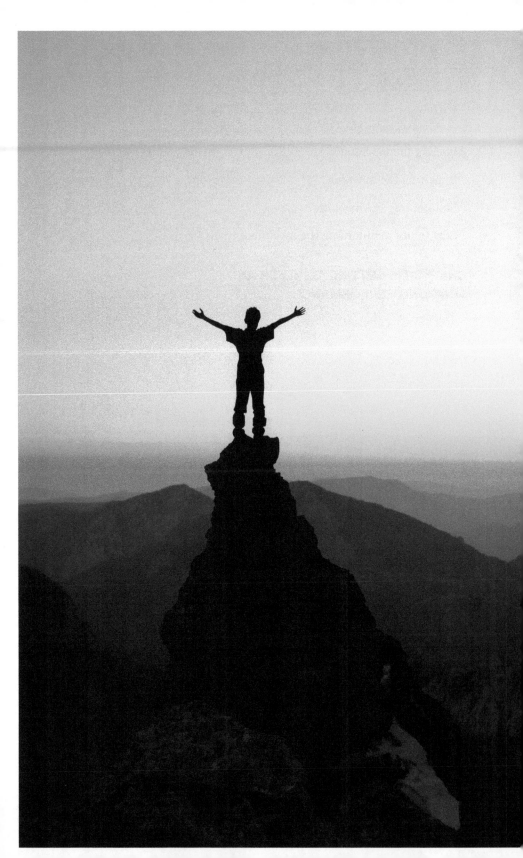

Introduction

One of my favorite experiences as a physician happened during a phone consultation about 4 years ago. It caused me to laugh out loud but, more importantly, it caused me to reconsider my standard way of consulting with clients. In my practice—at that time— most of my consults were in my office, face-to-face. Occasionally, however, my clients/patients would be too busy to come in to review their results, and set our next quarter's goals, so we would have the consult over the phone—this was one of those times.

Obviously this is not ideal, but I was quite comfortable with my ability to do this well, as I had done it many times before. I enthusiastically dove into a full review of all test results, comparing them to the previous quarter, discussing where we had met our goals and where we had fallen short. However, I was also going into great detail about my postulates for what physiologic changes had led to certain results and what our options were to test my postulate. I cannot recall how much (if any) verbal feedback my client gave me during my diatribe. But, about 30 minutes into the call he stopped me and said: "Doc, I don't need to know how the clock works, just tell me what time it is."

From that day forward I carefully looked and listened for clues that my client may not be interested in how the clock works. I had this lesson in mind in writing this book. In chapters 1-3 you will find a lot of information about how the clock works. You may not be interested in that information. If that is the case, feel free to skim and skip as you please, as the most important parts of the geeky information is repeated in chapters 4-9. Due to this approach there are a few redundancies in the book. For that, I apologize, but it was unavoidable in order to take the approach that I think will serve as many people as possible—by giving them the option to skip around the science parts, and come back to it if they please.

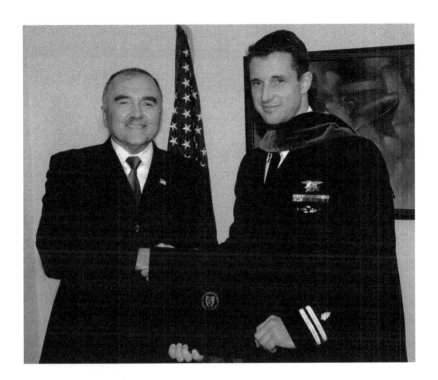

My Story

I was a successful power athlete for most of my life, never having any major health problems, just a few minor orthopedic injuries. I played football for 13 of the first 18 years of my life (in Texas, no less). I was a reasonably high-level competitor in track and field, powerlifting, multiple martial arts, beach volleyball, and crew. I am also a former Navy SEAL—which carries with it a substantial amount of mental and physical rigor. I have always found it easy to add muscle while staying fairly lean. I have studied nutrition to a reasonable extent, but I was never super-knowledgeable about diet--even though I often thought I was. I reached some pretty decent physical achievements this way, and therefore never gave much thought to lifestyle or diet. That is, until I entered medical school.

As anyone who has been there knows: medical school sucks! As a student, you are either studying, feeling guilty about not studying, or sleeping (while having nightmares about studying). I am a slow reader, so, as the volume of information increased, the hours of reading ramped up and the hours of sleep ramped down. After all, sleep is kind of a waste of time, right? Isn't sleep for the weak?

I was sleeping approximately four to five hours per night and rarely was it good sleep. I lived off of coffee and protein shakes. I simply did not have time to waste on cooking or going to buy food. So, I made three or four protein shakes every morning, and took them to school as my alternative to actually eating. The shakes were about 100 calories each. In the evenings, I'd have a fairly normal American dinner. On average, I was taking in about one thousand calories per day, and I weighed about 225-230 pounds. As you likely know, a guy my size needs more than double the amount of calories that I was taking in—just to not be wasting away.

Now you are probably thinking, How did this idiot get into medical school? Your guess is as good as mine. But, because I'm a hardheaded simpleton from the middle-of-nowhere, Texas, I decided that I would keep working out every day (at about 4 a.m. most days). Smart, huh? As I slept less and ate less, I somehow managed to get fatter. Much fatter! I was tipping the scales at about 240 to 245 pounds—and now (not so proudly) harboring about 18-to-20% body fat. I was no longer strong. I was no longer fast, and I certainly did not feel powerful. Ugly scaly patches began growing on my head—soon I would learn that I had developed psoriasis. My blood pressure increased about 20 points systolic, and my once perfect lipid panel began to evoke memories of Lipitor commercials. To take me down another level, my hair starting thinning, and my cognitive capabilities were in free-fall. Keep in mind all of this was happening at the grand old age of 32.

A year later, I was diagnosed as having ADD. I pretty much considered ADD to be a made-up crock of you-know-what just to get some prescription-quality stimulants. Unfortunately, stimulants did not help me much, so I rarely took them. Much later, I would discover that my change in attention was due to sleep deprivation—and the subsequent hormonal changes that this book will discuss.

Astonishingly, I made it through medical school and a year of internship. I would love to tell you that I achieved this after solving the riddle of my downward spiral, but I would be lying. I "made it through" ONLY because I didn't completely crash and burn before my training ended—although I was dangerously close.

Soon after escaping hospital rounds, but still sleeping only 4-to-5 hours per night, still undernourished, still flabby, still stupid, and still using topical steroids to control my psoriasis, I went back to the SEAL teams. This time as a physician.

To the surprise of many people, SEALs aren't just physical studs, they are smart. Really smart, and they have no problem questioning their doctor's knowledge. There is no B.S.ing them. They also operate on a system of pure meritocracy. If you are not up to the task, they will call you out. Then they will tell all of their friends that you are incompetent, and you will very quickly find yourself completely marginalized. I knew first hand it would do me no good to talk the talk if I couldn't walk the walk. To be successful in this environment, I'd need to be sharp, hardworking, and fit.

Again, I'd love to tell you that I solved the riddle in order to "fix myself," and then shared by discoveries with others that were facing similar challenges. What really happened—for the first time in over a decade—I had more time to sleep, as I no longer needed to go to the gym before or after work. My office was literally in a gym. My sleep became longer and of better quality, and I started eating better—because I was HUNGRY! I also started making fitness gains.

Encouraged, I carved out some of my spare time to study further. I studied a little about nutrition, a little about exercise, and a LOT about sleep. I also had the luxury of now working with some world-class trainers (Zack Weatherford and Josh Evert). Having been a SEAL in my early 20s, I assumed that things would be the same as when I left the teams (about 15 years earlier) and I would be doing a lot of sports medicine. This was my first big surprise of the job!

It quickly became evident the reason the vast majority of my patients came to see me was for the same reason that the vast majority of them were listening to Robb Wolf's podcast. As he puts it, "The wheels were falling off!" They weren't recovering well, their performance was diminishing, and their sleep had been terrible for years. But, like me, these guys just put their heads down and ran harder—sleep or no sleep—whether they felt like it or not. It was an expected part of the culture. That is exactly what we expect SEALs to do.

I once read a quote that went something like; "A professional is someone who does their best work when they don't feel like it." By this definition, I challenge you to find a more professional organization in the world. I have been in a few "elite" organizations, but no ne of them hold a candle to the SEALs. I will always consider any SEAL my brother, and my primary responsibility as a physician.

Therefore, I figured my number one responsibility (as their physician) was to figure out how I could get these men to sleep. Reason being I suspected lack of sleep to be one of, if not the primary reason, that the wheels were falling off. Given the culture, this is not an easy task. In Hell Week during SEAL training, we go a full week without sleep. Then when assigned to a SEAL team, we frequently sleep-deprive ourselves for days on end. So, my most immediate task was simply to get the SEALs to value sleep.

Medical school had not prepared me for this type of work. I do not remember a single lecture about sleep during any of my classes.

I also did not have any questions about sleep on any of the three licensing exams required to become a medical doctor.

My internship in OB/GYN had certainly not prepared me for this. Matter of fact, that's a profession where sleep deprivation goes with the entire career. My extensive sports medicine and orthopedics training had not prepared me for this job, and the common medical algorithms were of little use.

Figuring out why an entire community of elite performers, especially one this large, were almost all suffering from the same sleeping difficulties was not going to be an easy task. The reason for their predicament certainly was not from a lack of awareness, a lack of medical advice, a lack of funding, or from a lack of access to medical expertise. As I said earlier, these guys are smart, motivated, and at the top of the food chain.

Sadly, after making significant headway in helping my community, I have come to learn that much of the world suffers from these very same issues, oftentimes equally as severe, but usually just a little later in life than the patients I was treating.

Throughout this book, I will outline my discoveries of, and my approaches to, the absolute metabolic mess underlying our current national epidemic of inadequate sleep. I was facing a nebulous problem as to why these elite performers were suffering from the symptoms that usually plague men twice their age, and who were not nearly as fit as these younger SEALs, and I was the only one they trusted with their truth. After a lot of interviewing these guys, and a whole lot of research and self-guided education, I postulated that poor sleep was causing metabolic and hormonal derangement and that nutrition, lifestyle modification, and supplementation could correct these derangements. Especially sleep.

I hope that you will both benefit from and enjoy the information that I have compiled to address the dangerous epidemic of sleep deprivation that befalls us today.

My Basic Approach to Medicine

When you graduate medical school, they tell you that half of everything they have taught you is wrong, that it's up to you to figure out which half, and that the "wrong" half is going to change on a regular basis. We were told that we would be continually learning incorrect or incomplete information, even though we would be learning the best researched and most accepted information and theories available at any given time.

Since highly credible researchers commonly contradict one another, and it is often years before the argument is settled, I like to go back to what we call an "evolutionary biology model." This means go back to what you KNOW, as far back as you can. We know biochemistry, we know general physical chemistry, we know anatomy, we know physiology. These fields haven't seen many major changes in decades, and they are not likely to, at this point. These are foundations. So, anything you base off of these foundations, we say has biological plausibility. "It makes sense." It's a common sense kind of test.

The evolutionary component of that is basically this: we evolved a certain way, just like everything else on this planet. We evolved to be on this planet, and we evolved to succeed on this planet. So let's try to figure out what it was we were doing better, that was allowing us to be a part of this planet, before we completely took ourselves out of the planet's evolutionary matrix.

Yeah, I said it. If you really think about it, we have taken ourselves out of the evolutionary model. We make it dark when we want it to be dark, we can make it light when we want it to be light, we can cool our environment when we want it to be cold, or heat it when we want it to be hot. We eat whenever we want. We eat whatever we want. We reproduce when we want to reproduce, we grow fruit in the winter, we can do whatever we want. For all practical purposes, we have taken ourselves off the planet. As undesirable as that seems it appears to be working out pretty well, right? I'm not complaining. I'm not getting chased by a tiger and neither are you. We're at the top of the food chain, but there is a price for all we have accomplished.

So, I have re-educated myself in medicine. I have reconsidered and reframed everything that I learned in 10-plus years of education through an evolutionary perspective.

It's from this reworked perspective that I will talk about sleep, hormones, nutrition, exercise, reproduction, immunity, health and longevity. Most of what you will find in this book can be found elsewhere within the medical literature, in psychology literature, in health and wellness information, and in the general media. As I said, this is an evolutionarily-based approach. I did not invent evolution. I am part of it, and so are you.

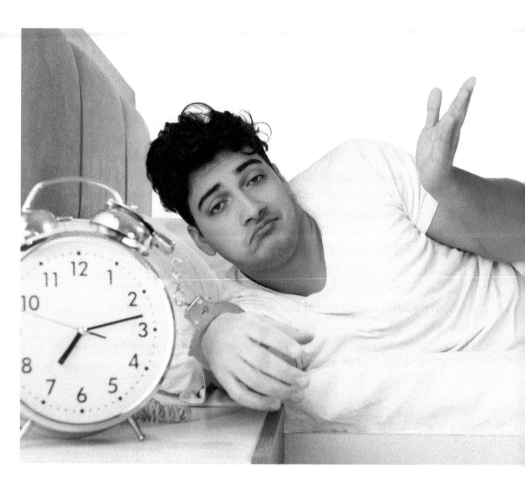

CHAPTER 1

What is Sleep?

Defining a tricky and complex concept

What IS sleep? What does it mean to sleep? Call me old-fashioned, but I think when learning anything, I need to begin with defining what I am trying to understand. So, let's start off with an easy question: What is sleep? We have all had the experience of sleep. If you haven't, please call me immediately because I would like to write up your case for the medical journals.

Think about it. It's actually kind of hard to define the concept of sleep. How can it be that something we all do every day is almost impossible to define? Well, I don't want to get too esoteric before you have had adequate time to judge my credibility, but here goes. Language is only an approximation of experience. And being an approximation, it makes certain things hard to describe or define. By and large, language is dualistic or comparative. For example, the word "big" needs the concept of "small" to make any sense, just as "up" needs "down," "right" needs "left," and so on. I digress. Don't throw the book away just yet. I'll try to stay on track a little better—back to the definition of sleep.

My favorite definition to describe sleep comes from the Dalai Lama of sleep research and sleep science, Dr. William Dement. It actually requires a two-part definition:

"A barrier between the sleeper and awareness or consciousness exists, and the 'sleeper' has to be able to overcome this barrier to become awake, when the environment requires it (such as machine gun fire, noises of burglary, and crying babies)."

My only addition to this definition is that you should have some reasonably predictable brain wave patterns (EEG). My reason for adding this part is due to the use of sleep drugs. As I will discuss later, if you sleep using sleep drugs your brainwave patterns will not look like the normal brainwave patterns associated with sleep.

We have all had the experience of falling asleep when we were not supposed have fallen asleep, whether you were working a nighttime security job, or on guard duty in the military, or in a classroom during a lecture. The interesting thing is that the smallest little thing can wake us from that sleep. But we will all agree that we were asleep. We know what the sensation of sleep is, an d we know that we were asleep. Conversely, especially the men, when you go to sleep in your own warm, safe, bed and somebody crashes their car into the front of your house, you might not wake up until your wife yells at you 20 times, and hits you with a cattle prod.

We can all agree that in both cases you're asleep. In both cases there's an environmental barrier, but that barrier height changes depending on what level of sleep you're in, how comfortable you are, how sleep-deprived you are, and so forth. Notice that the second part of Dr. Dement's sleep definition is that you can be awakened. So, with that part of the definition in mind, being in a coma or passing out from alcohol are not the same things as being asleep. If we can agree to use the two-part definition above, we can get started.

This is a good enough way of explaining sleep, since we all have had the experience of sleep. We already know about this barrier that exists between our environment and our conscious thoughts, and we can recall being awakened out of this state. If we cannot be awakened, we're either unconscious, in a coma, or dead.

The reason it is so difficult to define sleep is because there are hundreds of changes and reactions in your body that need to happen before you actually go to sleep, hundreds more to keep you asleep, and yet hundreds more before you can wake up. So, while the definition listed in the top of this paragraph may be accurate, it is incomplete. If you encountered someone who speaks your language, but has never had the experience of sleep (again, call me immediately), the previous definition would not suffice. A second definition and perhaps a more complete definition of sleep (for this book) uses the advantage of our dualistic language: **To be asleep is the absence of wakefulness.**

Now you're screaming inside of your head,'That doesn't mean anything!'You are probably thinking that this is a rhetorical definition. Stay with me a little longer. The reason I call this the most accurate and complete definition is because we do not actually have a proactive, sleep-forcing, biological system. What we do have is proactive biological system that forces us to be awake and aware of our environment—to the extent that our environment requires our awareness and interaction. For example, you will become much more awake at the sound of gunshots than the sound of the wind blowing loose shutters around.

This second definition lets us include the accurate but incomplete definition while adding some more meat to the concept, and meat—as we will talk about in a later chapter—is good. So, if you will allow me to use this rhetorical definition of sleep, we can proceed to some more satisfying information. Let's talk about that proactive system that drives wakefulness.

What governs wakefulness and sleep?

Wakefulness is governed by what we call our adrenal system. Notice I use the word system. I will use this word because other organs in your body control the adrenal organs, and the adrenals are responsible for effects in every tissue in your body. So, talking about the adrenals by themselves does not tell nearly enough of the story to get my point across. What do I mean that the adrenal system governs wakefulness?

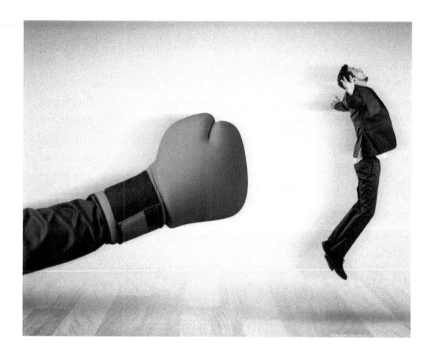

The flight-or-fight response

A lot of you may know that the adrenals control what Walter Cannon coined the "fight or flight" response. Most of us that have experienced the phenomenon of fight or flight would all agree that this is the most awake you can possibly be. You'd have absolutely no chance of dozing off while being chased by a tiger! If we can agree that this state is about as far away from being asleep as possible, then we have some solid footing from which to leap into the meat of this book.

I wish I could explain everything you need to know to understand sleep without using any scientific jargon. However, I am not yet a talented enough teacher to do so. Consequently, you will have to grind your way through at least some of it—if you want to know how the clock works. I urge you to set aside enough time to get through this first chapter, and I promise it will all be easier soon. By the time you have read these first three chapters, you will likely know more than your doctor about sleep, and you can teach him or her how to correct his or her own sleep issues.

Like anything else, improving your sleep requires an understanding of the problem. It is just like your diet. You need to understand which foods are detrimental to your health, and which foods improve and support your health. Likewise—if you understand what should be happening—you will be able to understand which of your behaviors are supporting your efforts to sleep, and which behaviors are hindering your ability to sleep. Thankfully, just like nutrition, once you get on a reasonable plan, maintenance is pretty darn easy.

The all-powerful governing hormones

The Adrenals:

The adrenal glands are two little anthill-shaped lumps that sit on top of your kidneys. As I alluded to earlier, these guys play a major role in making you feel and behave in ways that we associate with being awake. They do this by secreting many hormones that then go on to change the actions of all the other tissues in your body—collectively these hormones are oftentimes referred to as stress hormones. Now, as you might have guessed, your adrenals themselves don't have any way of knowing what your environment is. If there is a burglar in your home, your adrenals have no way of directly sensing it. They get help from your other organs; namely your eyes, ears, skin receptors, and brain. However, even in the absence of your eyes, ears, skin receptors and burglars, your adrenals can still wake you up, on cue, every morning.

How they do this is not precisely understood. The adrenals have a rhythm to them that are somewhat similar to the tides. The tides come up and go down every day on a rhythm. We know that this is caused by the earth's rotation and the gravitational pull of the moon. However, we don't really know what causes gravity. Likewise, the daily rhythm of your adrenals are associated with the rise and setting of the sun. (This is our first problem as modern humans: living with electricity.)

The entrainment of adrenals to sunlight is as good of a place to start as any. You have probably heard the term circadian rhythm. Like most scientific words, the word circadian has its origin in Latin: circa means about, and dia means day. So, circadian simply put is: about a day. This is accurate. In complete absence of any light, your circadian rhythm will run about 23.5-24.5 hours. However, defining the word that describes the observed phenomenon does not impart any more understanding. We must go deeper.

Retinal Ganglia:
Your eyes are a big player in this game. They actually sense the light, and they tell the brain what they are seeing. Actually, seeing isn't the right word. More accurately, your eyes tell the brain what they are sensing. Your brain then interprets what these sensations are most likely to mean, and then your brain alters your behavior accordingly. In addition, your eyes have a group of nerve cells in your retina called retinal ganglia that specifically sense blue light—presumably because the sky is blue. I can't be sure, because I was not involved in the design—but it seems plausible. This is where our story of losing the biological drive to be awake actually begins: decreasing blue light to the eyeballs.

Thousands of years ago, when humans were developing into the creatures that would harness electricity, build machines, and create the Cinnabon, we developed the ability to sense the sun's light, and the absence of the sun's light. We likely have never been well adept at seeing in the night time, nor have we ever been fast enough, strong enough, or lethal enough to compete with most of the planet's nocturnal predators. So perhaps it was a simple case

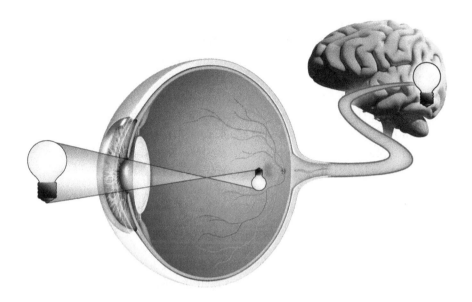

of natural selection. Perhaps the humans that felt awake at night
fell off of cliffs, fell into holes, or got eaten by big cats. However,
it's just as likely that humans have always been stimulated awake
by the sunlight, and in the absence of it, and began to feel sleepy
when the sun went down—due to the cellular functions that
combined to make us complex creatures. Which brings us back to
the retinal ganglia.

Step one: As the sun goes down, the amount of light entering
your eyes obviously decreases. More importantly, the amount of
blue light will decrease and be gin pushing you toward the process
of going to sleep. Notice that I said process. We like to say things
like "out like a light," but I can assure you that there is nothing
nearly as simple and absolute as a light switch involved in the
sleeping process. Hundreds of things must happen before we go to
sleep, hundreds more to maintain sleep, and even hundreds more
before we are able to wake up. The decrease of blue light on the
retinal ganglia is the first step.

Step two: The retinal ganglia increase their firing rate and begin to change the chemical composition of our brains.

Little structures called neurotransmitters control much of the activity of our brains. Just as their name implies, they are literally little signals, carrying messages from one neuron (a.k.a. nerve cells) to the next. Think of them as the much-folded notes that got passed around the rows of students in grade school. The students are neurons and each note is a neurotransmitter. The notes could cause an increase in activity (excitatory neurotransmitters) with a message like, "Ms. Jones has cookies behind her desk" or decrease activity with a message like "we only get the cookies if we are well-behaved today" (inhibitory neurotransmitters). Some kids are severely gluten-intolerant and may therefore display very different behaviors than the other kids who read the note. This is also true with neurons: some neurons are excited by a certain neurotransmitter, and some are inhibited by the same neurotransmitter.

The retinal ganglia stimulates the release and production of many neurotransmitters and neuromodulators. One of these neurotransmitters is known as GABA (gamma-amino-butyric-acid). Another important neuropathway eventually excites an area of the brain called the pineal gland (pronounced pie-neel). The pineal gland sits in the back of the brain and has been called the third eye by some more ancient and esoteric cultures. When stimulated to do so, the pineal gland secretes one of the most well known sleep enhancing hormones: melatonin.

Melatonin:

Melatonin then leads to other chemical cascades that decrease the secretion of stress hormones from the adrenal glands, those little organs sitting on top of your kidneys. Our adrenal glands secrete many hormones; DHEA-Sulfate, cortisol, aldosterone, epinephrine and nor-epinephrine. (If you're a geek like me, you might find it cool that epinephrine and nor-epinephrine are what we call " adrenaline " in common language because they come from the adrenals). Adrenal hormones control lots of stuff in your body, and when these hormones are really high, we call that " the fight or flight " response, which works great to keep us safe in really dangerous situations.

But in day-to-day life, the adrenals are designed to just keep us awake and alert in proportion to the environment we find ourselves in—which can occasionally be fight or flight.

Once adrenal function decreases, the effects of these adrenal decreases include the lowering of body temperature, a decrease in heart rate, and a decrease in blood pressure, slower neuron firing, lower blood glucose levels, and the we eventually fall asleep.

Of course, that's a whole new ball game.

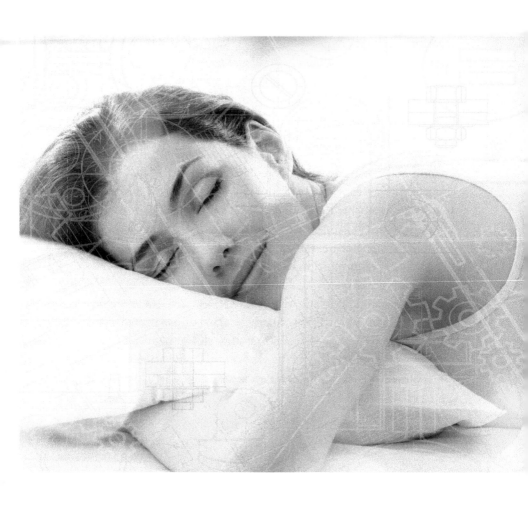

CHAPTER 2

The Mechanics of Sleep

Circadian rhythm

So you're probably beginning to get the picture that there's a lot going on within the mechanics of sleep. There's a great deal more to it then fluffing a pillow and turning out the lights. Indeed there is, and perhaps the more you know about it the more you will appreciate the complexity and why things like diet, exercise and sleep hygiene practices can have terrific impacts. So let's start off by talking about one of the most impactful influences on being awake and being asleep: adrenal hormones.

You've probably seen curves drawn on a chart (like the one below). These are NOT charts of daily cortisol levels, but represent adrenal function in general.

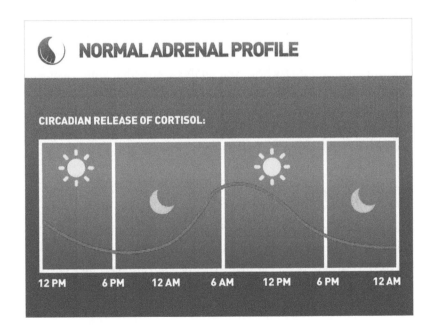

NORMAL ADRENAL PROFILE

CIRCADIAN RELEASE OF CORTISOL:

| 12 PM | 6 PM | 12 AM | 6 AM | 12 PM | 6 PM | 12 AM |

As I've mentioned, this is often referred to as a circadian rhythm. Circa means about, and dia means day, so it's a day rhythm, like the tide. Up and down, up and down.

This graph approximates cortisol, but it could be used to approximate many other adrenal hormones. I chose cortisol because it is easy to measure, it stays in the blood stream a long time, and it's a big molecule. Cortisol also has multiple measurable effects, but the one we like to talk about most is its ability to raise our blood glucose. It is in a group of compounds known as glucocorticoids.

In the picture above, cortisol is in arbitrary units. At some point in the picture above, your cortisol level goes down below the level that woke you up. Your adrenal function has decreased because the sun has gone down. After the sun goes down, you start feeling really sleepy. At the lowest part of the curve you are in the deepest levels of sleep—known as stages 3 and 4 of sleep (see the picture below). Stages three and four sleep are called deep sleep. This is also what we call "slow wave sleep cycles" (SWS).What is happening during deep sleep is the secretion of growth hormone and testosterone, which implies increased anabolic activity, or growth. When we are young, everything is growing, and this growth is obvious. After puberty however, anabolic growth mainly means repair; repair of overused muscles, injuries, brain tissue, and so on---- but only if cortisol is low enough. If adrenal function remains too high, a common problem in Western civilization, this anabolic period is compromised to some degree.

Normal sleep

Chronically elevated cortisol also beats down inflammation, meaning it shuts down the normal inflammatory response. If you have ever heard of people who have transplant surgery, they have to take a drug that is very similar to cortisol, in order to prevent rejection of the transplanted organ, because glucocorticoid

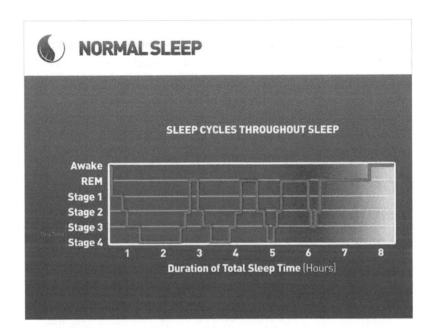

(cortisol-like) drugs essentially minimize your immune function—with long-term exposure.

More hormones

DHEA: Dihydroepiandrosterone (you can see why everyone just says DHEA) is another adrenal hormone. To be accurate, DHEA can be produced in other organs of the body. DHEA can go on to make testosterone, estradiol, or more cortisol. It can actually affect the nuclei of individual cells to help with energy production, thermal regulation of cells, and lots of other things like that.

Your adrenals also secrete a hormone known as aldosterone. Aldosterone lowers your blood pressure. Some forms of hypertension medications take advantage of this mechanism to lower blood pressure by acting like aldosterone.

Finally, I'll mention epinephrine and norepinephrine. These two hormones affect your blood pressure and also (through a different mechanism) your heart rate, dilation of your lung passages (bronchial tree), your attention, and lots of things that we can think of as being part of the fight-or-flight response or even a mild stress response.

When epinephrine and norepinephrine are in you bloodstream, we call them hormones. If they are in your brain, we call the neurotransmitters. That is why I say they can affect your attention. In fact, just to be a geek, I'll point out that they can affect your effect!

Connecting dots to insulin resistance

Hormones convey information throughout the body. Hormone sensitivity is the key to proper cellular growth, repair, and functioning. Almost everything that happens in your body happens can ultimately be traced back to hormones.

Additionally, what makes you feel better or feel worse has everything to do with hormones. It may be true that you have an intracellular (inside the cell) excess of so me form of protein or mineral. It may be true that your cell is failing to do this or that. It may be true that a cell is doing too much of this, but it's failing to do that or doing too much of this instead of that. But all of these are just the outcomes of what the hormones instructed the cell to do. Take insulin as an example. We know that people who have problems controlling blood sugar are called diabetics, and most people at least know that diabetes has something to do with insulin. If the cells of your body take insulin inside of the cells, this changes the machinery inside of your cell to also let glucose into your cells. However, insulin also controls how many receptors your cells have to bind insulin. So, if insulin has a hard time getting into the cells (because few receptors exist). We call this "insulin resistance."

Ironically, this lack of intracellular insulin will also result in fewer insulin receptors. It is easy to see how this self-perpetuating cycle can get out of control. In this example your cells would also get little glucose—which cells need to do their job, and you need as a fuel reserve. Interestingly, sleep deprivation in KNOWN to cause this same pattern of insulin resistance.

So, in summary, we can see that the adrenal hormones are increasing your blood glucose, affecting your heart rate, respiratory rate, blood pressure and metabolic rate, and affecting your attention, mood, focus and other cognitive functions.

It doesn't require an advanced degree in science to extrapolate how all of this might impact the fight-or-flight response. The fight-or-flight response will be an ongoing reference point in this book. I am sensing that your science tolerance gauge is entering the red zone. Let's switch gears to discuss something more pragmatic.

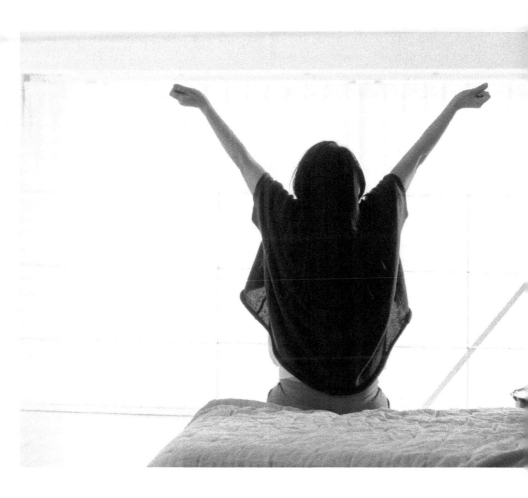

CHAPTER 3

*Optimizing Sleep
for Performance*

Optimizing Sleep for Performance

I get a lot of questions about sleep, as you can imagine. There are several key questions that deserve good answers. Let's take these on now.

How much sleep do you need?

For example, a patient will discuss his or her problems with me, and when I suggest improving sleep as a possible tool for reaching our agreed upon goals, they always come up with some version of "how much sleep do I need?" While this isn't quite a philosophical question, it is nebulous. My answer is always the same. "It depends."

If your goal is to survive, I cannot tell you how much sleep you need. There is too much biodiversity and too many variables to even approach this question. If your goal is to thrive, we have a place to start. Unfortunately though, all sleep is not equal, and you won't always need the same amount. For example, if you do not have any sleep debt (a concept I'll discuss later), and you have been lying around a spa in Fiji all day, you'll need less sleep than if you have huge sleep debt and you've just spent a 14-hour workday landscaping.

I should probably define the term "sleep debt" before I use it too many more times. I learned the phrase for Dr. William Dement—truly the grandfather of sleep medicine. It is a metaphor for understanding our sleep needs. Just like using a credit card, or a line of credit, you can spend money that you don't actually own. You can also operate you body on energy that wasn't intended for such use. The exact details of why we sleep are still not understood, but we all know it to be a restorative process. We knew that before anyone ever developed a test tube, a polysomnograph (sleep study), or discovered the first hormone. However, research is gradually confirming and better defining the restorative processes that occur during sleep. Keep in mind however, even if we can discover and define every process that occurs while we are sleeping, that information still may not explain why we need to be asleep to accomplish these processes.

One way to understand sleep debt is by looking at financial debt. For example, if you spend $5,000 per month, and you only earn $4,000 per month, you will be accruing a financial debt of $1,000 per month, for every month that you hold that pattern of spending. We all agree that at some point this pattern of spending will become unsustainable, and we will be in big financial trouble.

Likewise, if you need eight hours of sleep per night and you only sleep six, you are incurring a sleep debt of approximately two hours per night. The cells in our bodies do not run off of 24-hour clocks that we have invented to keep track of our perception of time, but they do have cellular mechanism in them that approximate the notion of time—so that is why I say "approximately two hours" of sleep debt. Just like with the overspending of money, at some point you are going to have to pay back the energy deficit that you have accrued by not allowing the body to restore itself fully—each night. It may not be until you go on vacation, or stay in bed for three days with the flu.

If you do not pay it back with sleep, your body will use resources that are meant for other activities (building collagen in your skin, building muscle, fighting off infection, repairing damaged tissue, etc.), to keep you alive and moving. This is equivalent to spending your child's college savings to finance your daily life. You may notice that the few examples of the consequences of not sleeping enough—listed above—are all things that we commonly associate with aging. That is not a coincidence. Sleep debt accelerates aging.

However, I will make a case for how much sleep most people need, on average, in order to avoid sleep debt. With the invention of the internet one can find data to support most any claim, but, most of the credible research supports that seven and a half to eight hours per night is the optimum sleep amount (keeping in mind that this is an average over multiple months). Dr. Dement, and others have done research in where they put people in completely darkened bedrooms for 14 hours per day, and the subjects would initially sleep about 12.5 hours for multiple weeks before gradually decreasing their nightly sleep to about seven and a half or eight hours per night. This process is called "sleep adaptation" which, in this metaphor would be the same as paying off that credit card completely.

There are lots of unanswered questions about the concept of sleep debt, such as, does it accrue linearly? How long can you carry a sleep debt? How can you distinguish sleep debt from organic disease that makes one sleepy? However, for our purposes, it is safe to say that if you wish that you could sleep more than you do, and you are sleeping significantly less than seven-and-a-half to eight hours per night, you most likely have some amount of sleep debt.

Exactly what is optimal sleep?

Optimal sleep has several components:

1. You should fall into it easily and relatively quickly. This actually gets into a concept called "sleep latency." We'll discuss this in detail later, but the basic concept is this: it should take you about 15 minutes to fall asleep. Substantially more or less indicates sub-optimal sleep.

2. It should be uninterrupted (or at least perceived as uninterrupted). Sleep studies reveal that we all wake up multiple times per night, but are usually unaware of this if our sleep is healthy.

3. It should be regular, meaning you go to sleep and awaken at approximately the same time every day, including weekends. There will, of course, be some normal variation to this with seasons, life stressors, and obligations. However, we are speaking in generalities here—an average over many weeks or months.

4. It should feel restful and restorative. THIS IS THE MOST IMPORTANT ASPECT OF OPTIMAL SLEEP! If you sleep exactly eight hours every single night (go to sleep and awaken at exactly the same time every day), and incorporate every bit of sleep information within this book, but you awaken exhausted every day, and count down the hours until you get to sleep again, your sleep is NOT optimal.

I will avoid going into a scientific diatribe on this question and just state some generalities. Everything that we need to repair is being repaired while we sleep. Your immune system can function at its maximal level (while you are asleep) because the adrenal function is at its minimal level. You consolidate important memories (we also clear useless information), whether that's remembering math formulas, phone numbers, girls' names, front-sight focus, overhead squats, clean-and-jerks, or playing the piano. Nearly all the stuff that we call muscle memory is becoming more embedded and durable during sleep. If you don't get optimal sleep your improvement and mastery of the skills needed to perform the skill you are working toward are greatly compromised. You can run through it every day of your life and, if you ignore your sleep, you are exceedingly unlikely become great at anything.

(As an aside, if you do want to become great at anything requiring muscle memory, I recommend Dan Coyle's book: *The Talent Code. For now, let's get back to optimal sleep.*)

Another thing that happens during optimal sleep is that you emotionally categorize the day's events. This single point has huge implications for the military, paramilitary, law enforcement, and any other type of emergency response workers. If you don't sleep well, then you cannot appropriately categorize events. You're much more likely to get post-traumatic stress disorder (PTSD). You are also much more likely to become an alcoholic, or dependent upon other drugs to decrease your anxiety and stress levels. You are even more likely to commit suicide. Let me write that one again: You are more likely to end your own life, intentionally, if you do not sleep well. If that isn't enough motivation to get you off the couch and into your bed, I cannot imagine what will be. Presumably, if you're more likely to commit suicide, then you must be more likely to become clinically depressed—since suicide is, by definition, nearly always associated with depression. You are also much more likely to engage in spousal abuse, child abuse, road-rage, and just about any other socially unacceptable activity one can think of. Why is this?

Remember when we discussed the little hormones in your brain called neurotransmitters? Well, these little hormones are not constant. They are constantly being depleted and restored. We replenish neurotransmitters during sleep—primarily during what we call REM sleep and slow-wave sleep. Not to be confused with the popular band in the 90s: REM stands for Rapid Eye

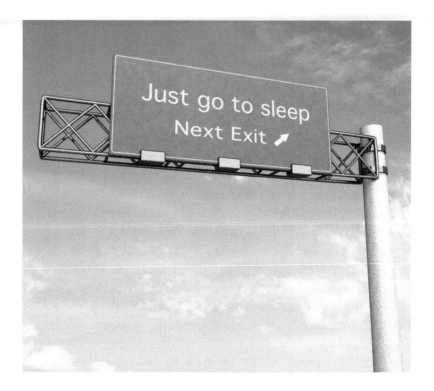

Movement, which was one of the first terms coined within the field of sleep medicine.

Optimal sleep is the sleep that makes you better; better looking and better at any type of activity—physical or mental. It allows you to become better at dealing with your emotions. With optimal sleep, you will be a better husband, wife, son, daughter, spouse, athlete, employee, entrepreneur, dancer, rapper, fighter, teacher, doctor, artist or whatever.

If you feel any of these aspects slipping, there is a possibility that not getting optimal sleep is part of the problem. It is possible that other problems exist, but if you know you are not sleeping well, this is an easy and necessary place to start looking.

How do you know if your sleep is optimal or not?

The most objective and easy way to get a read on the quality of your sleep is with a concept I introduced in the last section: Sleep latency.

Basically, sleep latency works like this: You do all of the stuff you need to do to get ready for bed—put on your favorite PJs, brush your teeth, floss, take your supplements, put on the heating blanket, turn out the lights, fluff your pillows, lick your elbows, or whatever your ritual is, and then you put your head on the pillow. (By the way, I will thoroughly discuss the importance of these types of preparatory behaviors a later in the book.) Once you're done with your ritual and you are actively engaged in the process of letting yourself "fall" asleep, the timer starts. Ideally (on average) you should fall asleep in about 15-20 minutes. If you fall asleep in less than 5 minutes, you are likely sleep deprived. A specific procedure of this measure is part of Dr. Dement's work and is referred to as the Multiple Sleep Latency Test (MSLT). A full MSLT is more involved than this, but this "time to fall asleep when you should be sleepy and when you should not be sleepy" is a reasonable approximation.

Next on my list of self-assessment is performance--in whatever it is that you do. A sudden decrease in performance, mental or physical, can often be traced back to poor sleep. I will discuss the actual hormonal changes later on, but let's just say you aren't firing off on all cylinders. This may be subtle: "I walk in a room all the time and I forget why I am there" or, "I often walk out to my car and realized I forgot my wallet." That kind of thing.

It may be not so subtle. "I go inside to get my wallet, I go back and get in my car and realize that I forgot my phone. I go back in my house, I get my phone, I go back and sit down and realize I forgot my briefcase ... 45 minutes later, I finally get on the road and start driving to work, I go past my exit because I'm going to my daughter's school and I forgot ..." and so on.

It may be severe and obvious: "I fall asleep on my way to work, I can't concentrate for more than 3 minutes, my FRAN time went from 3 minutes to 12 minutes, I've gained 15 pounds of fat but haven't changed my diet or exercise routine, I can't perform sexually, I cry during Hallmark commercials, etc.

Another signal that your sleep is suboptimal is chronic inflammation. I don't just mean that your joints are swollen or your eyes look puffy—while these are obvious outward signs. This is a metabolic condition that implies your body's cell-mediated immunity and repair is malfunctioning. Chronic inflammation happens because you don't repair at night. Your immune-repair mechanisms are malfunctioning because you have chronically elevated stress hormones.

Think about how you feel and function when you have the flu. Why do you feel like crap? Do you feel like crap because there's a virus in your body? NO! You feel that way because your body is fighting that virus. Your body is using much of the energy that it ordinarily uses to make you active and happy to fight that virus.

So, if you are chronically sleep-deprived, if you are not hitting those deep levels of sleep, and y our immune system isn't doing what it's supposed to do, then you're chronically inflamed. It is as if you're running around with 30 percent of the flu—every day.

To summarize, you should sleep at consistent and regular intervals, take 15-20 minutes to fall asleep, sleep through the night, and wake up feeling refreshed and ready to get out of bed.

How to become an optimal sleeper

The answer to this should be obvious. Just follow Dr. Parsley's easy 12-step process, and everything should be good in a couple of days, right?

My first comment to anyone that I consult on sleep is that sleep is an infinitely complex process. There are hundreds if not thousands of processes involved, all working in concert. There is no "easy button" here. It will require a systematic approach some trial and error, and some disciplined effort. This book will give you the framework to design your systematic approach. If you set about this process in a systematic and disciplined way, you will achieve optimal sleep.

One word of caution: please be realistic with your goals. I am as ambitious as anyone. I think lofty goals are the most inspiring, and the most likely to be achieved. However, you would not expect to lose 20 pounds in a few days, or go from a couch potato to being a world-class athlete in a few weeks. The more broken your sleep currently is, the longer it will take to perfect it. Remember, however, that you will begin to see improvements long before you reach optimal sleep, and once you achieve optimal sleep, you are unlikely to ever need to put much effort into it again.

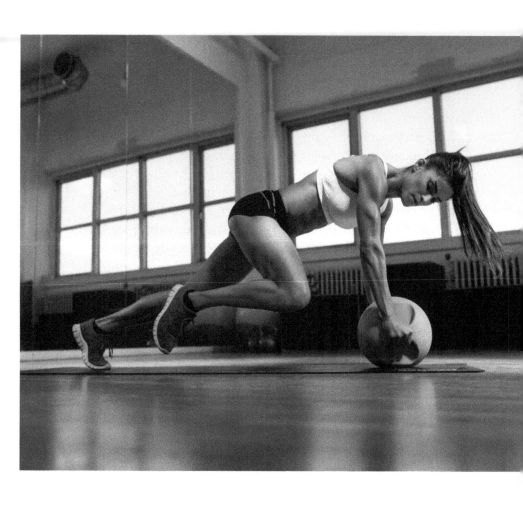

CHAPTER 4

Sleep and Physical Performance

Anabolic repair

I mentioned in earlier chapters that anabolic hormones are actually produced or triggered for production during sleep. While about 50% of the people that I talk to have heard something about this fact, few understand the magnitude of this reaction, and fewer still have thoughtfully considered the consequences of losing even a small part of this capacity. Hopefully, by the end of this chapter, you will be part of the unfortunately incremental population that understands the physical performance cost of even small amounts of sleep deprivation.

I would first like to clarify a term that is often thrown around in an inaccurate and prejudicial way:'Anabolic.'Most everyone has heard of anabolic steroids and when the word anabolic is used, it tends to conjure up an incomplete set of images. Unfortunately, due to sound-byte news and media hype, most people believe that anabolic steroids are a substance that athletes used to cheat in sports, or young men use to develop cartoonishly large muscles. While, those two perspectives are not completely inaccurate, they do lead to a warped perspective on what 'anabolic' means, a perspective that undermines why one might want to have more anabolic hormones floating around in their bodies.

The word anabolic is not in any way relegated to the development of muscles or athletic performance. Anabolic essentially means that there is a net increase in functional structure or activity in your body. Even more simplistically put, anabolic is the building up (repair) of your body and performance capabilities. The word catabolic means exactly the opposite. Rebuilding brain tissue, muscle tissue, liver tissue, connective tissue, and every other type of tissue is a net anabolic activity. The image of a lean muscular athlete is a fair representation of anabolic, while the image of a severely ill patient (perhaps a chemotherapy patient), or the disturbing images from WWII concentration camps, would both be accurate visual representations for catabolic. I want to emphasize this is a drastic oversimplification, but useful enough to keep the momentum of thought moving on this topic. With this visualization one can simplify a complex process into a fairly intuitive concept.

For a foundational example, adequate nutrition is likely to be (quite accurately) thought of as anabolic, while starvation would be catabolic. I will make the case that the most anabolic behavior that anyone can engage in is sleep.

As many of you reading this book probably know, we don't get stronger during the act of exercising. We make the gains and strength and performance when we are sleeping. Activity has the potential to simply maintain our capacity to not decay. Walking around the block for example will not turn anyone into a world-class athlete, but it will allow anyone to maintain a level of activity, on par with walking around the block, for as long as that person takes regular walks around the block. While this may seem fairly neutral, it is still an example of anabolic behavior. This is since all the universe is in continual decay (entropy), even the maintenance of the status quo requires net anabolism. However, I'd like to talk about actual growth—the growth of muscles to be able to generate more force, or sustain force for longer periods of time, growth of cellular organelles to allow that cell to live longer, or do its job better, the growth of synapses between the nerves controlling those muscles and cells, and the growth of the junctions where those cells meet their target. These are the elements of physical performance. So, when I use the word "exercise" it could be interchanged with "activity"— based on intention, more than outcome.

The concepts that I am about to describe apply to a growing child, a young adult trying to stay fit while starting her new career, a mother trying to maintain her ability to do the things that she loves to do—while still having energy for the kids. These concepts will obviously apply to anyone seeking to increase athletic performance as well, but I want to make it clear that anabolic is anabolic. What "physical performance" means is highly individualistic. However, the path to that physical performance is pretty darn similar for everyone.

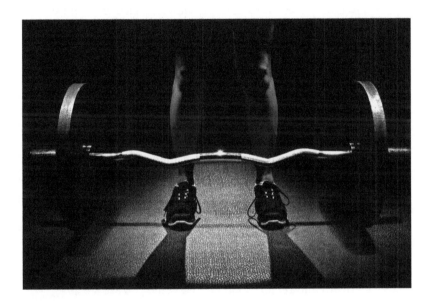

Sleep is repair

Let's get started. When we exercise, we are damaging the very tissues targeted for growth. For example, when you lift weights, with the intent of getting stronger, you're breaking down the muscles being exercised. We are consuming the fuel within those muscle cells and producing catabolic byproducts. We are also consuming stored and circulating nutrients to fuel the muscles. Ironically, the only way to get stronger is to heavily damage these cells. Cells need to be stressed before their performance will change. If someone does the same exercise, at the same intensity, with the same amount of nutrition and rest, at some point (regardless of how intense the exercise is—assuming your body can repair between workouts) this "exercise" would be more properly classified as an activity rather than exercise. Improvement stalls. In training and exercise circles this is commonly referred to as a plateau. On the other hand, if a person forces stresses and strain on their muscles and connective tissue, to the point that those tissues are not able to do their job well enough to keep up with the forces—a.k.a. muscle failure— then those cells will begin to adapt into a more robust form of themselves. They will make the necessary changes to be able to handle the stresses and strain placed upon them. The athlete will then place even more stresses and strain on those tissues. This might be in the form of more resistance as in adding weight to a barbell. Or the same amount of resistance but performing the work faster, within a decreased period. More speed, or longer durations of exertion, etc. More stress than the amount of stress that was previously applied. This is how we get physically better at physical activity.

Again, this is not an exercise physiology textbook. I am simplifying this process to get to my point, which is this: ALL of this anabolic growth and repair is happening while you are sleeping.

Slow wave sleep (SWS)

Deprive yourself of sleep, and you are depriving your tissues and cells of their ability to fully recover and improve. This is a point of the opening paragraph of this chapter. The growth, recovery, repair, improvements that I described require anabolic hormones to be readily available and catabolic hormones to be relatively low. Deep sleep (also called slow wave sleep, or SWS), is the most anabolic state. It is, in fact, the exact opposite of the phenomenon called "Fight or Flight." During fight or flight your body is actually using itself as fuel to get away from the threat. Energy is all that matters. Every function not crucial to fighting or fleeing stops. Stress hormones are at their highest possible production and secretion levels as well as their concentration. A key note here: Stress hormones are catabolic.

While we are in deep sleep, our bodies are repairing at the highest possible rate. Our brains are stimulating our endocrine organs to secrete the hormones we need to repair and grow. This includes testosterone, growth hormone, insulin, progesterone, thyroid and more. Our brains are doing this based off of what is floating around in our bloodstream and cerebral spinal fluid. Our damaged/fatigued cells are sending chemical messages to our brain to tell our brain that they are damaged. Our gut lining is sending these kinds of messages. In fact, any cell that is being challenged by bacteria, viruses, or parasite is also sending out these messages. Our brain is responding to our cells by triggering the release or creation of other chemical signals, secreting the precursors to the anabolic hormones needed for repair, mobilizing stored fuel, manipulating circulation, temperature, digestion, etc.

In other words, deep sleep is the time in your life when your immune system is functioning at its peak, your body's ability to repair is at its peak, and all resources for repair or immunological defense are the most available for every cell in your body.

Let's consider a practical example of this idea. Let's say you want to increase how much weight you can lift. This can be either a one-repetition life for maximum weight (a strength gain), multiple lifts over the same amount of time (primarily a gain in power), once over a shorter length of time (primarily a gain in speed). The only way you will reach your goal is to push the tissues involved beyond their present ability. After you have pushed those tissues past their limits (all cells involved in that activity/exercise) you must give those cells the nutrients that they need to repair (food). You must be in a hormonal and metabolic state that allows these tissues to repair and improve (sleep). Again I am being overly simplistic for the purposes of this book—since this book is designed to foster an interest in using sleep as a resource for performance enhancement, not coach the reader in his or her preferred sport.

SEAL Standards

When I was working as a physician for the SEALs, the guys that came into my office to seek advice about losses in physical performance almost always had one of three things going on: They either deprived themselves of sleep, or had great difficulty getting quality sleep, or difficulty getting sufficient sleep. They were frequently using presumed sleep aids (alcohol, anti-histamines, prescription sleep drugs, or a combination of these). When I looked at their lab test values, anabolic hormones where almost always extremely low for their age and fitness level. Their inflammatory markers and oxidative markers (both inflammation and oxidation are catabolic) were almost always extremely high. Interestingly, they would not have met the criteria to be diagnosed with any metabolic or endocrine disease. Not by Western medical practices, that is. Nonetheless, the SEALs have their own acceptable standards for performance, and if they fell below SEAL standards, it was (to the SEAL himself) synonymous to what a Western trained physician would classify as a "disease." The upshot was that Western medicine had little to offer these guys. Oddly enough, the limitations of the Western definition of disease, juxtaposed to what the SEALs considered acceptable performance to be, required me to completely re-educate myself as a physician.

I'm sure that you can guess the conclusion to this chapter's information and argument? Although, I would have never imagined it to be true or even likely at the start, getting these SEALs to sleep more, without sleep aids, very often led to a complete reversal of all of their performance concerns. They shed unwanted fat, they improved their speed, power, endurance, strength, and ability to recover. While I did employ supplements, there was no drug to solve their issues, there were no diagnoses that would help guide my treatment, and my medical education had provided me very little help in solving this riddle. Who would have ever guessed that some of the highest performing men in the world, Navy SEALs, men with a focus, drive and determination second to none, would be able to improve their physical performance to a level they hadn't experienced in a decade, simply by changing how they thought about and practiced the function of sleep? I was as surprised as anyone, and it was a long time before I was confident enough to stand my ground when being challenged by the naysayers. Equally surprising, I will now stand up in front of any size audience and declare with confidence and fortitude that sleep is absolutely, unquestionably, the most import factor in athletic/physical performance. I'm not saying that sleep alone is sufficient to become a better physical performer. I am saying that it is essential, and should be the seeker's highest priority.

Perceived Effort

The real challenge to the reader is not accepting what they have just read. The challenge to the reader is putting what you just read into practice, while being pressured by life-long beliefs, social constructs, ignorant coaches and leaders, and the ubiquitous claims of icons that they only sleep 4-5 hours per night. Most of the time I have found these claims to be dubious at best. However, even when a high performer has proven to me that he or she sleeps significantly less than what research shows to be optimal, when they are willing to listen to me and prioritize their sleep, even these high performers register enormous improvements in their performance.

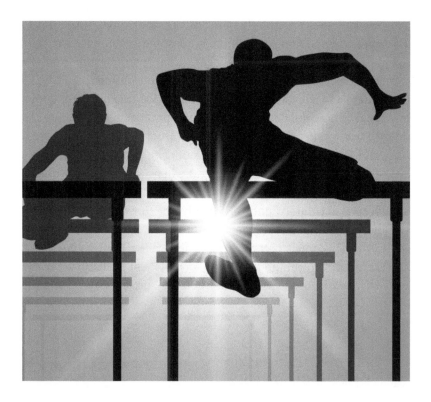

In a later chapter I will discuss cognitive performance in greater detail. However, I would like to close this chapter with the concept of "perceived effort." This term is pretty intuitive. It is the performer's subjective experience of how hard it was for them to execute the activity (i.e., how heavy the weight felt, how much pain did the activity cause, how hard did the performer have to push themselves to reproduce previous efforts. That kind of thing.). It is well researched and well documented that perceived effort can play a significant role in physical performance. It probably won't surprise you when I tell you that it is also thoroughly established that inadequate sleep is highly correlated to perceived effort. Every hour of sleep you short yourself leads to a noticeable increase perceived effort. So, think twice about joining that 5 a.m. workout group. Exercise, without adequate sleep to recover, is catabolic. It also seems harder and is less enjoyable, and is counter-productive to the performance gains being sought.

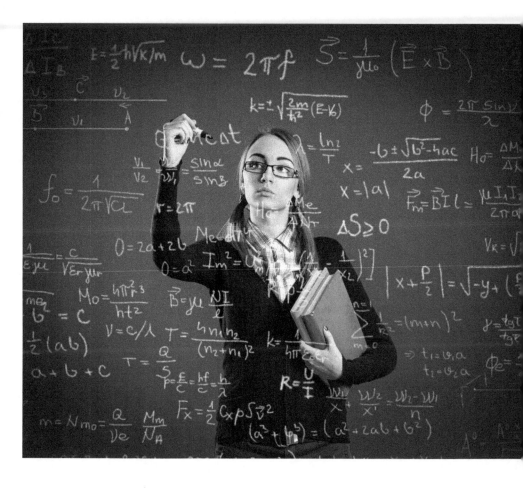

CHAPTER 5

Sleep and Cognitive Performance

Not an obvious correlation

As a physician that travels the world espousing the performance-enhancing benefits of sleep, I have discovered an interesting dichotomy. When I'm speaking to athletes—from college-level through to big-league professionals, Olympians etc.—they all seem easily willing to accept the idea that they recover during sleep, and that sleep is therefore at least somewhat important to their training and performance, but they usually balk at the cognitive and emotional benefits of sleep. Conversely, when I work with entrepreneurs, and C-level executives, they too are pretty willing to accept half of what I preach. Interestingly though, it's the same half that the athletes are willing to accept. One would think that a person who earns a livelihood almost exclusively through their decision-making capabilities, ability to learn, process, and work creatively with new information would recognize the detriment of poor sleep on their performance. However, such is not the case. Like the athletes they accept that sleep will help them with their triathlons, marathons, cycling, CrossFit etc., but they are often completely unwilling to consider the possibility that sleeping more would make them better at their job.

As perplexing as this may seem, the reason that this happens is obvious, once you learn about the behavior of a sleepy brain. If you have ever seen one of my lectures or TEDx talk, you will likely recall the simile that I am about to propose. There is an enormous amount of research dedicated to this very concept. The concept is self-awareness. In the last chapter I discussed how one's physical performance is diminished by inadequate sleep. The good news is that most people dedicated to some sort of physical performance have some metric for measuring their performance (timed with a stopwatch, how much weight, number of wins, etc). But, how does one measure their day-to-day cognitive performance? How do you know if you made good decisions today? It isn't as easy as measuring whether or not you netted the outcome you expected or wanted. Most real-life decisions have multifactorial inputs, outcomes, and an array of contextual interpretation. At first it may seem daunting to give an accurate measure of cognitive performance. However, some especially clever researcher figured out a way that has proven highly reproducible. It retrospect, it seems obvious—like most brilliant ideas. Most of the westernized world has experienced an altered state in which they either realize during that altered state, or after, they are no longer altered and that their cognitive performance is/was impaired. The state that I am referring to is intoxication with alcohol. As it turns out, one can pretty easily assess the cognitive functioning difference of a person before they consume alcohol, and that same person as they progressively drink up. The researchers can then correlate impairment with blood alcohol levels, and this type of research is what sets the threshold for blood alcohol limits for driving a vehicle on public roads.

Blood alcohol level

While we are a long way from being able to (and probably willing to) impose similar limits with sleep deprivation. As luck would have it, we can measure the same effect that sleep has on cognitive performance in a very similar way to how we measure the effects of alcohol. However, the level of total impairment (or impairment relative to one's optimal state) is not as clear cut as being sober from alcohol. Unfortunately, the "sober" base-line with sleep is somewhat laborious and time consuming. It requires the research subject to do what we call "sleep adaptation." This means the researchers take care of your entire life for you, and you lay in a cool, dark room for 14 hours per day, sleep as much as you want to, until you are consistently sleeping approximately the same amount of hours

per day. It surprises most people to learn that when this type
of research has been conducted, the average adult begins the
study sleeping about 12.5 hours per day and in 4-6 weeks ends
up sleeping about 7.5 hours per night. This is where the 7.5-8
hour recommendation originates from, and is the metaphorical
equivalent to "sober."Unfortunately, most of us do not have 4-6
weeks to clock 14 hours per day lying around sleeping.

Fortunately, this non-parallel does not completely
hamstring our ability to collect meaningful data on people in
the real world. As it turns out, we can still measure the effects
of performance decline and compare it to blood alcohol levels—
even without beginning the study with an ideally "sober" subject.
What we do is designate their "sober" with a base-line derived
from performance markers collected while the subject sleeps
what they normally get for sleep. I don't want to beat this to
death, but the nuance that I'm trying to communicate is that
the average westernized person is actually somewhat impaired
at their "base-line" because the average westernized person is
sleep deprived to some degree. Nonetheless, we can still use
their usual level of impairment as their base-line (for any type
of testing) and then measure how much worse they get when we
subtract from their usual amount of sleep. So, we are not able to
say how impaired they are from their ideal state, but we are able
to measure how impaired they are compared to how they started
the experiment (before we deprive them of any sleep).

The end result of this type of study, however imperfect, allows
us to compare performance declines from sleep deprivation to
performance declines associated with blood alcohol limits. If you
have ever been intoxicated, or had to deal with an intoxicated
person, you have probably noticed that self-awareness isn't a
strong suit of this brand of impairment. Being drunk doesn't
correlate with knowing you're drunk. I propose that the lack of
self-awareness that we associate with intoxication is the same
reason most people are resistant to the idea that their lack of

sleep is impairing their performance. In turn it makes sense that depriving one's self of approximately 2 hours of sleep leads to a performance decline on par with a blood alcohol level of .05 percent. However, if this person is sleep deprived 2 hours per night for 11 nights in a row, their performance decline (compared to their ideal "sleep adapted" self) is on par with a blood alcohol level of approximately .08 percent to 0.1 percent.

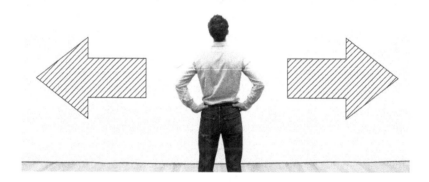

Baseline performance

Your objection is noted: "Why isn't all of the westernized world performing like they are slightly intoxicated on a daily basis? Since we know that the average American only sleep about 6.3 hours?"

I submit that they are. The problem with detecting it is that we consider the performance of a person that is chronically sleep deprived to be "normal." Our base-line measurement of "normal" is skewed. This same phenomenon can be seen with what we consider "fat" to be, or tall. One hundred years ago, six-feet-tall was very tall for an American. Today six-feet-tall is a pretty "normal" height. I don't know the numbers for body weight and amount of body fat, but we can all see the same progression with what we consider "normal" to be. It is therefore a completely rational argument to say that what we now consider "normal" cognitive performance to be would have been considered impaired 100-150 years ago.

I realize that is a pretty bold statement, but if you are not already in this kind of impaired cognitive state, I encourage you to remember a point in your past where you felt completely overwhelmed with information, a point where there was either too much to think about or too much information flooding in all at once. I pose this question to you: Why is there a limit on how much information you can process? The answer is pretty intuitive: Limited energy. I use the word energy loosely here. I use it to mean either the fuel for the neurons to fire, the substrates, neurotransmitters, neuropeptides and/or neuromodulators. The process of "learning" implies that the brain is altered in a way that allows the brain's operator to access information that was not previously accessible. The actual physiological and structural changes that occur, in order for one to learn, is way beyond the scope of this book. If you want to dig in on Google Scholar, by all means do. That said, I can list some very broad points if you are interested in knowing the general principles.

Brain energy

In the way I used the word "energy" in the paragraph above, I say the following: The energy state of your brain is extremely dynamic. It is literally changing by the millisecond. However, in the 'overwhelmed with information' memory I asked you to recall, the problem is that the brain is burning all of its energy to process what is already happening, and more information simply causes that energy to scatter. Once the energy is scattered, your brain then has to struggle just to get back to where it was before the new information was presented. Just imagine that you are drowning and a really attractive person is giving you his or her phone number. Of course there is no possible way that you would remember or even be able to pay attention to the phone number.

Your brain is doing everything it can to keep you alive. When you see, hear, touch, smell, or taste something new or different, when you think a thought that you have never thought before, when you try to imagine the likely consequences of your next decision or action, or when you compare and contrast information that you have never compared before, your brain requires energy—above its base-line consumption—to consider or learn this new thing.

Self awareness

You have probably heard before that the brain uses a highly disproportionate amount of our body's glucose supply. In fact, the brain—when viewed as a single organ contained within your skull—uses more energy than any other organ. What you may not know is that your brain's ability to function is also limited by the neurotransmitters, neuromodulators, inflammatory chemicals, waste products (from the brain's daily work), stress hormones, anabolic hormones, and many other factors. There is a limit to how many of any of these things can be produced and accessed by the brain. Can you guess what behavior plays a big role in dictating how much of this energy is available?

When we sleep, our brains actually flush out waste products known as neurotoxins. Our brains also balance out the neurotransmitters involved with being awake, learning, mood, communication, perception, and self-awareness. When we sleep, stress hormones are lower. Stress hormones inhibit your ability to learn. In the drowning metaphor above, your inability to hear or focus on the phone number being uttered by the attractive other is in part because your brain is overloaded with information, but that's just part of the deal. The primary source of overload are stress hormones.

Compounding fight or flight

If you have ever studied the "fight or flight" response to a life-threatening situation, you probably know that all of one's resources are being marshaled to keep the person a live. Any bodily function that does not contribute to getting away from the threat will go by the wayside until the threat is over. Evolution has prepared us for these types of threats, through trial and error. Hundreds of thousands of years worth of programming has led to some pretty predictable, innate, and reproducible actions during a life-threatening event. One of those predictable actions is a near complete shutdown of our big human brain (neocortex), specifically the regions of our brains that make us "smarter" than every other animal on the planet. Not thinking and being impulsive is actually one of the predictable behaviors I was alluding to earlier. Believe it or not, in most life-threatening situations that we evolved to encounter, it is better NOT to think your way out of it. It is better to be reflexive, impulsive, and highly action oriented. It is way better to focus on the threat than think about calculus, taxes, business, or even the attractive stranger on the shore.

This is probably not surprising. But, what if I told you that the same thing can happen under stress that is not of the life-or-death variety—to a lesser degree? Let me tell you what I mean. Let's give an arbitrary number to the amount of stress hormones and brain changes that involved in fight or flight. We'll call that a 10. Now, let's give an arbitrary number to the amount of stress hormones and brain changes associated with being awake, and living through a typical day for this 100,000-year-old body. Let's call that number 2 (Austin Powers joke). The nervous system (brain, spinal cord and nerves) controls the amount of stress hormones, and how much is perceived as a threat, and to what level. So, let's say that your boss or best client looks at you in a way that you perceive to be disapproving or angry. Perhaps a look that translates into a threat to livelihood? Maybe a letter from the IRS, an email from an angry friend, relative, customer, that kind of thing. These could all be perceived as threats. What about the idiot that is only 6 inches away from your back bumper while your going 75 MPH down the freeway? All the political and social unrest in America right now. We also tend to live in a continual state of response to demands. Bills, phone calls, texting, emails, meetings, traffic, information about how what we thought was healthy is actually killing us...

Average cortisol

The important takeaway is that any stimulus that we do not know what to do with or how to react to is registered within us as a threat. With that in mind, I think it's a safe postulate that our ancestors did not endure anywhere close to such frequent threats and potential threats that we do in modern times. If you'll follow me on that postulate, it's probably not unreasonable to assume that our stress hormones are higher (as in the sustained 24-hour average) than our ancestors. On our scale of 1-to-10, we need to be at a 2 for optimal functioning. What if, all of these constant stressors push us up to a 4? Our brains won't work quite as well, but we are nowhere close to the fight or flight. But, if we add sleep deprivation to that situation... BAM! The opposite of fight or flight (when your brain is actually repairing, pruning, getting rid of useless clutter, waste products, excess neurotransmitters—and solidifying useful information, rehearsing what you have learned, reliving salient events from the day, and increasing the neurotransmitters and hormones that you need to be at your best) is deep sleep. Sleep at night is repairing your brain from the day's events, and preparing your brain to deal with what's coming tomorrow. Excess stress hormones lead to poor or inadequate sleep. If we sleep poorly, our bodies then have to redirect more energy to operate our brains and bodies from somewhere else. Unfortunately, this process produces even more stress hormones. Remember the state of being catabolic we talked about in the last chapter? Stress hormones alter your physiology towards being more catabolic. Do you remember our visual picture for catabolic?

Excess cortisol

The important takeaway is that any stimulus that we do not know what to do with or how to react to is registered within us as a threat. With that in mind, I think it's a safe postulate that our ancestors did not endure anywhere close to such

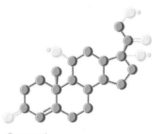

Cortisol
$C_{21}H_{30}O_5$

frequent threats and potential threats that we do in modern times. If you'll follow me on that postulate, it's probably not unreasonable to assume that our stress hormones are higher (as in the sustained 24-hour average) than our ancestors. On our scale of 1-to-10, we need to be at a 2 for optimal functioning. What if, all of these constant stressors push us up to a 4? Our brains won't work quite as well, but we are nowhere close to the fight or flight. But, if we add sleep deprivation to that situation... BAM! The opposite of fight or flight (when your brain is actually repairing, pruning, getting rid of useless clutter, waste products, excess neurotransmitters—and solidifying useful information, rehearsing what you have learned, reliving salient events from the day, and increasing the neurotransmitters and hormones that you need to be at your best) is deep sleep. Sleep at night is repairing your brain from the day's events, and preparing your brain to deal with what's coming tomorrow. Excess stress hormones lead to poor or inadequate sleep. If we sleep poorly, our bodies then have to redirect more energy to operate our brains and bodies from somewhere else. Unfortunately, this process produces even more stress hormones. Remember the state of being catabolic we talked about in the last chapter? Stress hormones alter your physiology towards being more catabolic. Do you remember our visual picture for catabolic?

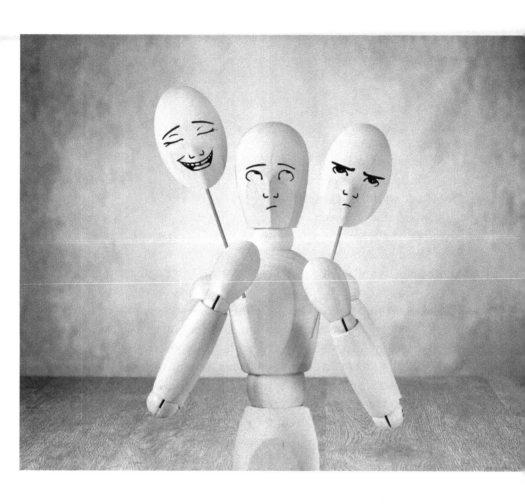

CHAPTER 6

Emotions and Mood

Why emotions change with sleep

Let's put this all together and into perspective. Excess stress stimulates the release of stress hormones. Excess stress hormones interfere with cognition. Excess stress hormones also interfere with sleep. Sleep is how we repair our brains, producing anabolic hormones, pruning useless information, and solidifying useful information. Our "usual" environment takes us from a basal stress hormone level of 2, up to a 4. Poor, or inadequate sleep pushes our stress hormones up a bit more (let's say to a 6). Which means our brains are operating at a level of stress that is about half-way to fight or flight. (where our brains are essentially uncontrollable). Once we are consistently operating at a stress level of 6, everything in our life seems a little more stressful, and we may even push up to a 7 or 8. At this point we say we are, "super busy." However, excess stress hormones are interfering with our ability to think, learn, communicate, process, schedule, focus, concentrate... and our ability to sleep well. Our sleepy stressed out brains make us much less productive (about 30%, less, if 6 hours of sleep becomes our norm), which means we need more time to get the same amount of work done. We perceive that work as more stressful. When we are stressed our mood reflects that, and we get less joy out of our work, obligations, and activities. Ironically, the only way to improve our mood, efficiency, ability to think, learn, and rebalance our neurochemistry is to sleep more.

I don't know about you, but I've marveled at how many times that the methods, practices or rituals that I am employing to reach a goal are actually the exact behaviors that are preventing me from reaching that goal. I slept 4-5 hours for about 12 years. Yet another example of youth being wasted on the young.

Couples study

A great example as to how powerful this effect is demonstrated is something called a couples trial. The researchers would take monogamous couples that reported a good/healthy/stable relationship and ask them to participate in a sleep deprivation trial. The basics of the trials were that one of the partners would sleep their regular night's worth of sleep, and one partner would be deprived of two hours of sleep. The upside was that the next day the partners got to spend the whole day together, without any of their normal responsibilities, and in some trials the activities they engaged in were paid for by the researchers. Sounds pretty ideal, huh? Be free of all responsibilities and go have a fun day with your significant other. On the house! At the end of the day they had one task. They were separated into different interview rooms and were asked a series of questions about their significant other. Essentially, they were being asked to rate their partner on how well he or she had performed as a partner on that day. They were asked about the communication, connection, emotions, and mood of their partner. By this point in the book, you think you know what I'm about to tell you, don't you?

Well, I have a surprise for you. BOTH partners rated the other as performing below their average. In other words, it didn't matter which partner was sleep deprived. It decreased the enjoyment for both partners equally. Both partners reported that their significant other just wasn't as present, as connected, as communicative, as fun, in as good of a mood etc. as they usually are. How can this be? I hate to do this, but I'm going to wax a bit philosophical again. Relationships are nothing more than communication—whether verbal, physical, non-verbal, body language, facial expressions etc. Any relationship is basically a sustained conversation. If you change that conversation, you change that relationship. When you impair one partner's ability to communicate effectively, the

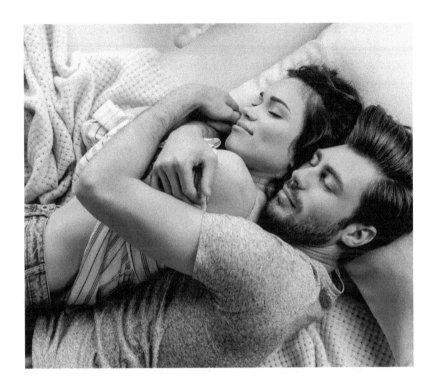

communication is worse. They both perceive it. They both report it, at the end of the day.

Since this is not a relationship book, you may be thinking, "So what"? Well, I challenge you to come up with a profession, goal, ambition, life-design or whatever you spend your time working towards and tell me that your ability to communicate will not affect that goal one bit. Even if your goal is to win a local age-group race; do you have a training partner? Will you have as much time to train if you cannot communicate well at work? Will you be in the same mindset to train if your personal relationships are strained? What about your communication with yourself—your inner voice. As your mood depresses, your self-talk becomes more negative, more judgmental, and less optimistic. Sleep deprivation makes you more anxious, too—due to the increase in stress hormones, and lack of mental clarity from inadequate brain repair at night. Also, if your goal is to run that race, go back and re-read the physical performance chapter—the part about all repair happening during sleep. But I digress ...

Sleep-deprived. Or ADD?

When we get inadequate sleep, we do not clean and prepare our brains well for the next day. Our neurotransmitters, neuromodulators, neuropeptides, and neuroactive hormones are out of balance. This literally leads to a measurable difference in brainwave patterns, and a measurable difference in PET scans and Functional MRI's of the brain. Your brain actually changes how it operates. Your brain will display a difference in blood flow to different brain regions, a different allocation of, and consumption of, glucose. Some regions of your brain that should be engaged, while you are engaged in an activity, will not be engaged—or will be to a much lesser degree. Additionally, brain regions that are not usually triggered by that activity may actually dominate the brain's functioning around that activity. The pathway that alerts you to danger will be much more active, regardless of the environment that you are in. The pre-frontal cortex (what Dr. Robert Sapolsky so cleverly calls our "simulator") will not be functioning. That simulator is your key to being your best self, regardless of what your goals are. That simulator allows you to weigh your current options—while considering your future goals. That simulator allows you to predict (as well as anyone can) the most likely consequence of the actions/decisions available to you. In fact, if you want to have some Kirk-like fun, look up the symptoms of attention deficit disorder (ADD), and then look up the symptoms of chronic sleep deprivation. With about 90% of our adolescent children being sleep deprived (due to school start times, and the circadian changes associated with adolescents),

I think we have to wonder if the epidemic of ADD in American children might be better explained by chronic sleep deprivation.

Anyway, back to my original point: if sleep deprivation and ADD are nearly indistinguishable (if you hadn't looked it up yet, sorry for the spoiler), ask yourself this question; "Would having ADD make me a more focused, emotionally stable and motivated person?" Would it allow you to feel more joy? Would it improve your mood? Would it improve your relationships? Of course not. That is why it is called a "disorder." Additionally, in the cognitive performance chapter, I wrote about learning, decisions, executive functions, etc. Do these things require the right mindset, the right mood, the right emotions, to perform your best? I de scribed how the fight or flight response shuts down your pre-frontal cortex. How well do you think you could communicate while being chased by a tiger? Or drowning? How motivated would you be sit down and chat with your wife and kids, discuss business ideas, design your training plan, read a history book?

Sleep is not a luxury

There is yet another aspect of how sleep deprivation affects our motivation specifically. Motivation, determination, will-power, and all similar descriptors of human behavior, are limited by our cognitive ability. Your prefrontal cortex has to be doing its job in order for you to take actions now that are designed to create a better future (delaying gratification). However, your brain is sort of like a switchboard. It is not only sending out signals, it is also receiving signals, and connecting various bits of your brain, based on the signals it receives. Unless you run a ketotic diet, your brain is using glucose—almost exclusively—as its energy source. When the signal comes in that your brain's glucose levels are declining too quickly (the total amount does matter—only the rate of change), your brain's perception is that you—as an organism—are at risk of starvation. Your brain then

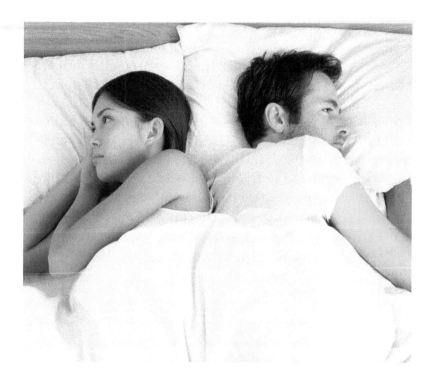

reallocates energy and blood flow to the areas of the brain and body that will protect you from starvation. As you might have guessed, your quarterly financial goal, your upcoming race, your job performance, your communication skills are not what your brain is considering to be essential functions to reduce the risk of starvation. Future direct motivation, emotional stability, mood, communication, are all higher-order brain functions. Just like your brain is unwilling to take in the phone number while you are drowning, your brain is unwilling to consider your future ambitions when it perceives that you are starving. The neurochemistry will simply not be in your favor. So, here's the rub: Insulin sensitivity and cortisol (think stress hormones) control your blood glucose levels. We've already discussed that sleep deprivation increases stress hormone levels. Would it surprise you to learn that insulin sensitivity is also drastically reduced with a single night of sleep deprivation?

Hopefully, by this point in the book, you are coming to the realization that sleep is not a luxury—indulged in by the weak, lazy, and non-productive. Not only is sleep absolutely essential to the optimal performance of every cell in your body, it is the most essential of all. If you are well rested and in good health, not exercising for a week or two is not going to have much of an effect on your physiology. You can also go several days without eating, and have completely normal cognitive functions. But, if you go several days (or weeks) without sleep, you will be broken in every way. Compared to most other animals on this planet, we are a pretty weak, slow, non-threatening animal. Our brains are what has placed us at the absolute top of the food chain. Our brains have enabled us to learn how to trap and hunt animals that otherwise could destroy us in a confrontation. Today, it is your brain that is allowing you to be a member of society. It is your brain that is allowing you to plan for your future. It is your brain that is allowing you to communicate with other people, to show and understand emotion, to set goals, prioritize and take actions toward your dreams. I've already shown you how a sleep deprived brain is similar in function to an intoxicated brain. In this chapter I've shown you how your sleep deprived brain is similar to a brain with ADD.

If you want to improve how you perform emotionally and professionally, if you want to avoid anxiety, stay positive, stay ambitious, and work towards the life of your making and your passion, would you think for a second that developing ADD and staying drunk all of the time would be helpful?

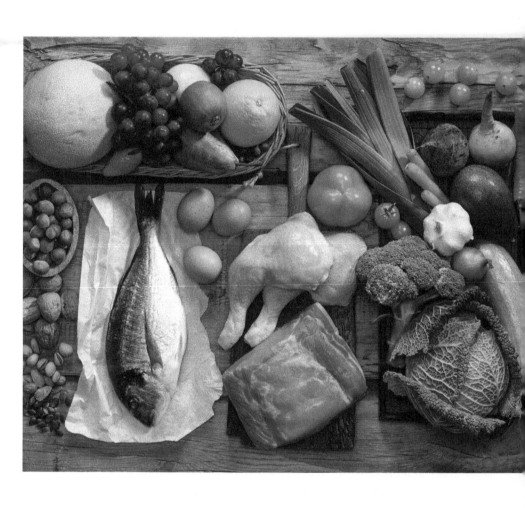

CHAPTER 7

Sleep and Nutrition

High performance machines

So far, in this book, I've been writing about sleep as the most important aspect of health. Yet I am often asked what I believe is the next most important aspect of health. My answer, today, is the same as it was in 2009 (when I first started lecturing about sleep). The answer is nutrition. I'll get a little geeky about exactly why in minute, but first, I'd like to offer a metaphor to simply the concept, and then we can get into the weeds about the mechanisms that drive the relationships of sleep, nutrition and performance.

I'm kind of a car nut, and always have been. My first car was a canary yellow 1973 Mustang. If you follow me on social media, you may have seen a picture of my son's first car, a n olive green 1973 Mustang. So... not much has changed in that aspect of my life. It was Peter Attia who got me interested in Formula One. If you've never had a thing for F1, I implore you to go online and google "F1 vs. Café racer." If that doesn't impress the hell out of you, I don't know what will. F1 cars are such an incredible feat of engineering that it is literally incomprehensible to me—even though I've been tinkering around with performance cars my whole life. These cars are capable of ground speeds that are mind bending. They can corner so fast that the lateral G-forces involved are beyond what the average car nut could even withstand. In fact, most of us could not even drive an F1 car, even though we've been driving our entire adult lives. These cars have to be driven fast enough to meet the engineering design of them or they simply cannot be driven. They are engineered in a way that causes the air pressure, created by going fast, to push the car into the ground hard enough to increase the traction on the wheels. Essentially, going really fast makes the car heavy enough to corner like it's on rails. If the driver isn't capable of driving the car fast enough, the car isn't capable of going around corners at high speed—because there is not enough air pressure on the car. Additionally, the acceleration and speed that these cars can reach is far beyond what would be expected by a car enthusiast that understands horsepower to weight ratio. These are essentially fighter jets on the ground. But, since I don't know anything about fighter jets, I'll stick with F1.

At this point, you may be wondering what the hell F1 cars have to do with sleep and nutrition. My answer is not much. I went into such detail to give you an appreciation (and comparison) of how amazingly these machines perform. There is literally nothing on wheels that can match the performance of these vehicles. They are the most performant vehicles in the world. They have evolved significantly, and quickly, over several decades. Humans have evolved over millions of years to be the most performant animals on the planet. No other animal is even close to our capabilities. Our nearest primates can't even build a grass hut, or write a sentence, or plan for the future.

Fueling the machine

So, if we use an F1 car as a metaphor for a human, I can point out some ideas that will seem pretty obvious—when applied to a race car—but, for some reason, not as obvious in comparison to ourselves. I'll start with a little hyperbole. If you owned an F1 car, would you use kerosene as fuel? No? Would you use 87-octane pump gasoline from Costco? If not, why? This is completely obvious when we apply it to F1. But, humans think they can starve themselves, or eat processed foods that their bodies were never designed to use as fuel, an d still perform well. If you owned an F1 car would you instruct the driver to never come into the pits? Not possible right? Why? The obvious answer is because, if the car does not go in for pit stops, it will run out of fuel.

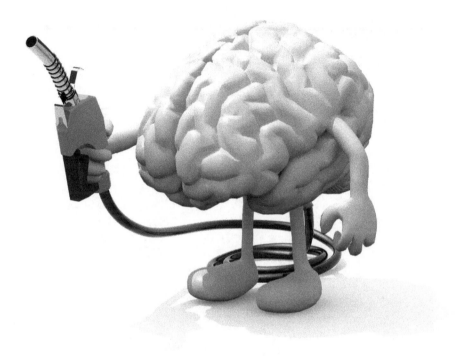

Repairing the machine

But, what else do they do in the pit stops? Change tires, make
minor repairs, make adjustments to fit the stress on that particular
day, with that driver, on that track. Humans also need pit stops.
We need to fuel our bodies, we need to make adjustments to
the stresses of that day, in our current mindset, with that day's
physiologic stress.

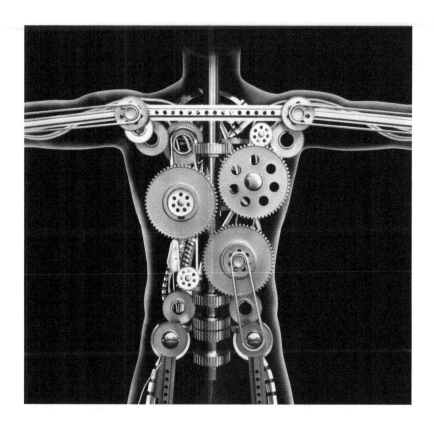

Maintaining the machine

Finally, if you owned one of these multi-million dollar machines, would you instruct your crew to cut corners on all repairs? Would you tell them to do just the bare minimum to maintain the car? Would you tell them to ignore any new technology that will make your car faster and more likely to win? How would you chose your driver? Would you just ask your next-door neighbor to drive for you—as a favor—or drive it yourself? You obviously own this thing for the purpose of getting the highest return on your investment, and therefore the highest performance you can get out of the car.

Why don't we treat ourselves that way? Why do we not marvel every day at the complexities and performance capabilities of the human mind and body? For, as amazing as F1 engineering is, as complex as they are, for all of their awe inspiring performance—they were created by humans. We are actually orders of magnitude more complex, more highly engineered, and more capable of awe -inspiring performance. Yet, we often treat ourselves like a cheap econo-box car that was designed as the bare minimum of what we expect a car to do.

In this metaphor, the repairs and upgrades that I discussed are a metaphor for sleep, and the pit stops a re a metaphor for lifestyle. Fuel, of course, is a metaphor for nutrition. Again, it is completely obvious in this metaphor that you cannot ignore any of these aspects, when we frame it as performance related to a car. If you ignore any one component, it is completely obvious that you will be subtracting from the car's performance. The exact same is true for our brains and bodies.

Cost in not maintaining the machine

As per usual, I have to say I am over-simplifying the rest of this chapter, in hopes of giving you a digestible overview of the relationships between sleep and nutrition and performance. Robb Wolf is a dear friend of mine. If you don't know who he is, you should definitely put his name into Google and go to his website. Robb's message is primarily nutrition, but he also talks a lot about sleep. I first met Robb while we were lecturing at the same event, and I was quite surprised by how much he talked about the importance of sleep. He was hired to speak as a nutritional expert. Likewise, he was surprised by how much the hired "sleep expert" was talking about nutrition. The bromance started immediately and continues to this day. In fact, Robb was a major contributor in helping me get my sleep supplement (Sleep Remedy) to the market.

So, let's get started. I think most people reading this book would likely accept the concept that what a person eats and how much a person eats will have a large impact on how their body looks (fat- to -muscle ratio) and performs. I wonder, however, how many readers think the same about nutrition and cognitive performance, or nutrition and sleep? I also wonder how many readers realize that what a person's body does with the food consumed is every bit as important as what food that person eats. Would you believe me if I told you that sleep is essential in determining what you want to eat, how much you eat, and what your body does with what you eat? If that seems like a stretch, hopefully this chapter will convince you otherwise.

Let's start with what you have chosen to eat. Have you ever noticed a difference in your appetite when you are sleep deprived? If so, have you ever wondered why this change happens? Well, the exact biochemistry and neurochemistry is beyond the intention and scope of this book, but here are the basics. When you do not get enough sleep—as we have discussed—it alters your neurochemistry. I have not written much about how it affects your body's chemistry and physiology, but it has equally damning effects. For instance, a single night of a two-hour sleep restriction results in about a 30% de crease in insulin sensitivity (how well your body responds to the hormone insulin), in multiple tissues of your body. One of the tissues affected is your subcutaneous body fat (the fat we see in mirror). Most people don't know this, but fat is part of our endocrine system (hormonal system). Fat cells secrete a hormone called leptin. Leptin then goes to a region of your brain that monitors your blood for numerous things— including hormones. One of the hormones that it monitors is leptin. Leptin is essentially a signal to your brain that lets your brain know how much body fat you are carrying around, or more accurately, how quickly are you using body fat as a fuel source.

Since body fat is meant to be a fuel storage tissue, the brain will make adjustment to other hormones to make sure that your body doesn't run out of fat (stored fuel).

The adjustments that the brain makes to your hormones and nervous system then determine how hungry you are, and to a large degree, what type of calories you are craving. When we are sleep deprived, our fat cells do not respond as well to our insulin levels. If they are not responding to insulin well, that is essentially the same physiologic state as having less insulin than we need. As we discussed earlier, insulin is a big fact or in regulating our blood sugar, and our brains rely on blood sugar as fuel. When we do not consume enough food, our blood sugar levels decline. Our brain and body perceive this as possible starvation and start responding in ways to make up for the lack of food. One way that our body makes up for our food deficit is by mobilizing our stored fuel (glycogen and fat). I know this is getting geeky and convoluted, but trust me. It will make sense in a second. Just hang in there a little bit longer.

If we are sleep deprived our fat cells behave as if we are underfed (because they perceive insulin as being low). They then send the signal (leptin) to the brain, to tell our brain that they are sacrificing themselves—for the greater good. Our brains do not need insulin to use glucose, so the brain itself may not be perceiving any deficiency in fuel. So, now the monitoring system of our brain (hypothalamus) is getting mixed signals. On the one hand, the fat cells are telling the system that the body is starving. On the other hand, the brain is sensing normal blood sugar levels. Just like in life, mixed signals are stressful, and our brains respond as to stress by signaling our adrenals to secrete more stress hormones. Those stress hormones then signal the tissues in our body to increase the available fuel for the body and brain. As we talked about earlier, one way to increase the available fuel is by increasing the catabolic activity of our cells (breaking big structures into smaller parts). However, another way to increase available fuel is to consume more fuel. Our bodies can use our stored fat pretty well as their fuel. But fatty acids cannot get into the brain, so our brain still really wants more glucose (carbohydrates), but our brain also knows that our body is using its fat cells as a fuel source. The result of all of the shifts I've detailed here is that we start craving sugar and fat. I believe this is the primary reason that doughnuts and other breakfast pastries exist. Our brain is also tired from our lack of sleep (since the brain's chemistry is rebalanced during sleep) and we therefor need to block the chemicals in our brain that are making us want to go to sleep (adenosine). Caffeine blocks the receptors that bind to adenosine in our brains. Now you understand why coffee and doughnuts are so common, and if you think of the late night shift-working policemen, it makes that stereotype pretty obvious.

This is just one example of how sleep restriction/deprivation affects how our brains and bodies process the environment they are presented with. The super-high glucose levels and insulin response, associated with eating doughnuts, have their own pathways to further encourage eating more of the same kinds of foods, but I will not get into that. That is more in Robb Wolf's and Peter Attia's lane than mine.

Another example of the relationship between sleep and nutrition is found in the lining of our guts. In the medical world, everything from your mouth to your anus is considered one tube (mouth, esophagus, stomach, intestines, colon etc.), and inside of this tube is actually considered to be outside of your body. What you put into your mouth has to be absorbed through the lining of the tube at some point, to be "inside" of your body. If we damage the tube (leaky gut) or change the way the tube decides what to let inside of us (gut biome), then we affect which elements of what we ate actually gets inside of the body. You can probably guess what I'm about to tell you. Sleep deprivation leads to increased inflammation (swelling

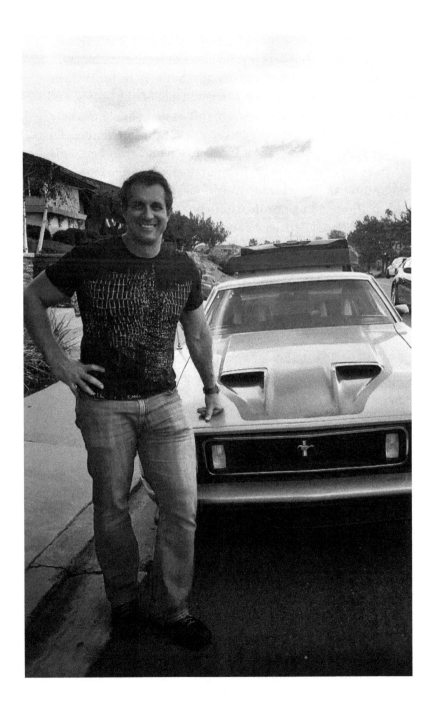

and immune system actions). Leaky gut begins with chronic inflammation. Sleep deprivation also effects our gut biome. Our gut biome are the bacteria in our gut that help us break down our food into molecules that can get inside of our bodies, and shield the lining of our tube from things that should not be getting into our bodies. When you change the gut biome, you change how the food you eat is processed and absorbed. This can have a profound effect on micronutrient and macronutrient absorption, an d can lead to nutritional deficiencies that then lead to other derangements within our physiology. Oftentimes those nutritional deficiencies can lead to catabolic activities in our bodies and brains.

Yet another factor to consider is that the sleep deprived brain does not work nearly as well and—as discussed in the chapter on cognitive performance—one of the primary regions in the brain that suffer from sleep deprivation is the pre-frontal cortex. Since this region of our brain is our "simulator," we are likely to care less or underestimate the physiological consequences of poor food choice. Also, the prefrontal cortex is essentially the region of your brain that is associate with willpower. If your brain's and body's physiology is screaming "starvation," the immediate solution to that starvation will overcome your best intentions.

As an interesting aside, the only time that any animal on this planet (other than humans) purposefully sleep deprive themselves is when they are starving. When an animal is starving, it needs more hours per day to look for food. It also needs to be more willing to try novel foods. Since avoiding starvation is their primary focus, their brains are also willing to accept more risk to get food. This is what leads to animals coming out of their normal environment into ours (our environment would usually be perceived as too risky) and eating out of trashcans. Interestingly, these same behaviors—sleep deprivation and risky behavior, not eating out of trashcans—can be observed in sleep-deprived humans. It does not matter if your body is actually starving or if your metabolic markers/signalers/hormones are presenting an environment consistent with starvation. In other words, sleep deprivation causes physiologic changes that are perceived as starvation. The perception of starvation leads to worse food choices and more food cravings. If you do not cave to these poor food choices, the starvation signals will increase. When the starvation signals increase, you will begin having difficulty sleeping. And, as we've discussed, sleep deprivation will make your brain think that you are starving.

With inadequate sleep, you will choose worse foods, you will crave more food and crave worse -food choices and your digestive tract will not be able to extract as many nutrients out of your food. Your poor food choices, and the chronic inflammation associated with sleep deprivation, will cause your gut lining to leak things into your blood stream that should not get in there. This will also lead to changes in which foods your gut biome can deal with (by changing the dominate bacteria in the gut). All of these things will lead to nutritional deficiencies. No machine can perform optimally on the fuels that it was not designed for—including you.

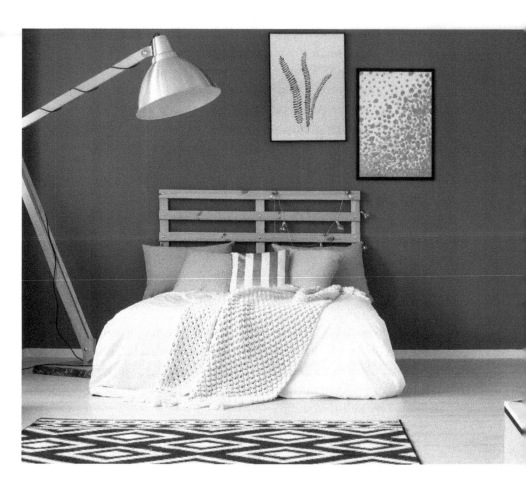

CHAPTER 8

*Getting to Sleep and
Tracking Performance*

2+2 always equals 4

As I continue to work with clients and patients over the year, the most common question is something like,'How can I keep my suboptimal sleep patterns and have optimal performance—in other words, can you make 2 plus 2 not equal 4?'The answer is obvious. However, I realize that there is a distinct difference between ideal and realistic. If you have an hour commute to work, you're a single parent, and you have a home-based business—just to make ends meet. I understand that you probably can't afford to make a whole lot of changes to your schedule, and you—of all people—need to perform optimally. You are the type of person that keeps this country going. Sometimes it's a first responder, an ER physician or a law enforcement officer on shift work. Or maybe a military combatant. Obviously, these people have little control over when and how much opportunity they have to sleep. So, the question posed at the beginning of the paragraph is a valid one. Unfortunately, there is no substitute for sleep. If it were possible to have optimal performance, optimal health, optimal longevity and sub-optimal sleep, through some kind of trick, hack, or magic pill, I would be first in line. The grim reality, however, is that if you do not sleep optimally, you will not be able to perform optimally in any area of your life. But, we can mitigate the detriments to your performance, health and longevity. There are dozens (if not hundreds) of little changes that will improve your performance, and decrease the impact of your sub-optimal sleep. There are some nuances, and complexities, to exactly how you string them together. To get the maximum performance available to you, you will likely need to work with an expert in the field of sleep and performance. Unfortunately, there are not that many of us around. Yet, anyway: Keep checking back with me on my site, as I am trying to build a network of such experts, and may possibly offer a coaching certification in this area—in the near future. The good news is you can probably get 80% of the way to your performance goal without an expert, and with some rigorous research and self-study, you could likely get another 5-to-10% performance boost.

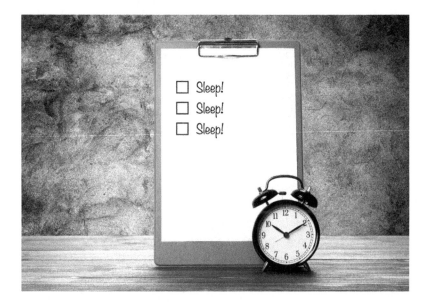

Prioritizing sleep

Nonetheless, there is one thing that every single person pursuing this personal performance enhancement MUST do. The unavoidable requirement for getting the best sleep, recovery, energy, mood, and performance that you seek is to first accept the reality that sleep is the most important aspect of performance for every person on this planet. Nothing will break you faster than poor sleep, and nothing will enhance your performance better, fast, or more consistently than getting optimal sleep. If you can accept this fact, internalize it, and live your life accordingly, we are ready to move on. If you cannot accept this fact, then go back to the beginning of the book, and start over, or do more research on the cost of poor sleep. Once you are ready to admit that sleep should be your first lifestyle priority (yes, I'm saying it's more important to get an extra hour of sleep than to get an extra hour of exercise, or an extra hour of work, or an extra hour with your kids), you are 50% of the way to your best possible performance. I make this bold statement based on many years of working with private clients. I have seen a pattern. Most people can intuitively figure out about half of the solution by merely being focused on the intention to get better and more sleep. Conversely, you can understand all of the science around sleep, mitigating behaviors, hacks, tricks, supplements, etc., but if you focus on those instead of earnestly pursuing the best sleep possible first, you will never reach your full performance potential. I think I have beaten that point into the ground, but the rest of this chapter is fairly useless without one's declaration to prioritize sleep as number one.

Sleep hygiene

The first step to optimizing your sleep and understanding any of the many tools to improving your sleep is to understand the concept of "sleep hygiene." You can access thousands of opinions online about the criteria for proper sleep hygiene. However, instead of trying to memorize the list, or becoming neurotic about following certain steps every day, I find it most helpful (for my clients and patients) to explain the concept of sleep hygiene, and the intention behind the criteria behind the list of acceptable behaviors. As I said in the beginning of the book, our bodies have evolved to use the sun as our primary cue for when we should be awake, and when we should be awake. When we study cultures that have yet to be exposed to electricity (yes, there are still lots of people that live the way we evolved to live) it takes an average of 3.3 hours, after sundown, before they fall asleep. The reason for this is that lots and lots and lots of changes that must occur in your brain before your brain and body will be ready to change— but the changes do not happen if the blue light from the sun (or light bulbs, TV's, computers, smart phones, etc.) is still radiating into your eyes after sundown.

So the first problem is removing blue light. This essentially means most light. Additionally, one of the many changes in your brain is the increase in the amount of a neuropeptide called GABA (after lots of other shifts occur in your brain). This happens gradually over the course of the 3.3 hours that we evolved to transition into sleep over. GABA has many functions, but one of the functions is to slow down the neocortex (aka cerebrum). This is the part of the brain classically shown as a human brain, one illustrated in pictures and cartoons of the brain. This part of the brain sits on top of (and sort of straddled over) what is often referred to as our "lizard brains." It is called the lizard brain because it is the part of the brain that even the least evolved animals on the planet have. In academic circles this part of the brain is a combination of the midbrain, brain stem, and spinal cord. This is the "unconscious" or "subconscious" region of your brain. It is performing functions that we do not intentionally have to think about; breathing, heart rate, blood pressure, digestion, etc. Obviously we need this region of our brains to keep working while we sleep. So, the function of GABA is to slow down our use of the neocortex, yet leave the lizard brain functioning at full capacity. All of sleep hygiene is aimed at addressing one or both of these conditions, as in decreasing blue light into your eyes, or slowing down the neocortex.

The practical application of sleep hygiene has been right in front of us, for our entire lives. If you've ever had kids, or if you've ever been a kid, you will remember that there is a "bedtime routine" to get a kid to sleep. If you have any experience with small kids, you know that it would be a completely unrealistic idea to let a 3-year-old kid rough house, and bang around with toys or games, right up until bedtime, and then pick him or her up and put him or her directly into bed, in a dark room, and then walk out of the room. We know that the ideal way to get the little monster to actually stay in bed and go to sleep is through a protracted ritual. We gradually limit their activity (in the hours before bed time), then we give them a bath (which lowers their body temperature slightly—another cue for sleep), then we put them in some soft snuggly PJ's, add some water absorbing, and even softer, powder to their bodies, then we get them into the bed—with some light still on. Next we start distracting their busy little brains by telling them or reading them a story (slowing down the amount of activity required by the neocortex). Then, we give them a bit of affection (laying with them, snuggling with them, hugging them, kissing them, etc.), which future reduces their stress hormones. Finally we assure them that we are going to be really close to them, and we will come to help if they get scared, and turn out the lights.

Compare this to the lifestyle most of us execute, in particular how we plan for bedtime. Most Americans (and other westernized citizens) tend to have more work, more obligations, and more obligations on top of those, and more things on our "to -do list" than we can possibly get done in a day. We frenetically shift from one task to the next, or try to multi-task (which research shows isn't even within the capacities of the human brain), and very often we are racing the clock to get one more thing done before bedtime. My experience with high-level executives, techies, entrepreneurs, and busy mothers is that they literally do this right up until they collide with bedtime. They actually climb into bed with their minds racing about what they haven't finished on that day, what they need to get done tomorrow to make-up for today's shortcomings, what mistakes they've made today that led to them not finishing everything they wanted to get done, or the work that they were finishing right before bed. This obviously violates the second principle of sleep hygiene—the slowing down of the neocortex. Our neocortex is how we interact with the world. All of our perceptions are processed in this part of the brain; what we see, what we feel, what we hear, what we taste, how we feel about all of those perceptions, and what those perceptions mean.

I find that most people can relate to my favorite example of this type of behavior interfering with our sleepiness. Have you ever woken up in the morning so exhausted that all you could think about is how soon you can get back in bed? You resolve to come straight home from work (or other obligations) and go straight to be d, so that you can "catch up" on your sleep. Then, one of your friends talk you into going to happy hour. You've been tired all day at work, you are still exhausted when you leave work, but you agree to go for just one drink, and then you are going home to sleep. After your second or third drink—a Central Nervous System depressant, which should make you feel even more tired—you are fully awake, feeling great, and determine that you don't think that you really need to rush home to go to sleep. You feel prepared to just get 6 or 7 hours and pop out of bed tomorrow. So, what happened? Did your brain "recharge" somehow? No, your brain simply had a lot of stuff to focus on, a lot of things to perceive—interesting conversation, funny jokes, loud music, television sin every direction, and attractive people that you might like to meet,. In this case, even if you had worked by candlelight for the past 3 hours, all the while wearing blue -blocking glasses, and were in a darkened bar, and therefore had the optimal amount of GABA in your brain to do the right things to prepare your brain for sleep, you consciously overrode the benefits of the GABA by stimulating your brain. This stimulation released additional stress hormones to keep you alert in proportion to the demands of your environment. Working right up until bedtime, worrying about the days events when you get into bed, planning for tomorrow's challenges (or mulling over today's events), has the same effect as the happy our scenario.

If you follow these two concepts, you can probably create your own bedtime ritual and sleeping environment, without any outside help. However, Google "sleep hygiene" if you feel the need, and you will find myriad ideas and practices that are designed to take advantage of these two concepts.

Sleep environment

The next thing to consider (still technically part of sleep hygiene) is your sleeping environment. We should associate our sleeping environment (bed and or bedroom) with only one or two things: Sleep or sleep and sex.

For the sake of clarity, I am not saying that you should only have sex in bed. I am saying that the only things that you should do in your bed are sleep or have sex. It's not the place for important conversations, reading, emails, social media, gaming, or watching TV (some of these, of course, violate the concept of removing light from your eyes). Also, as I mentioned earlier, one of our natural cues for sleep is a cool environment. Ideal sleeping temperature is actually around 64-68 degrees Fahrenheit. Your environment also needs to be quiet, feel safe, and comfortable. Remember that anything in your environment (or brain) that requires your attention will override GABA and increase stress hormones—both of which interfere with the quality of your sleep, and your ability to fall asleep (and therefore sleep duration).

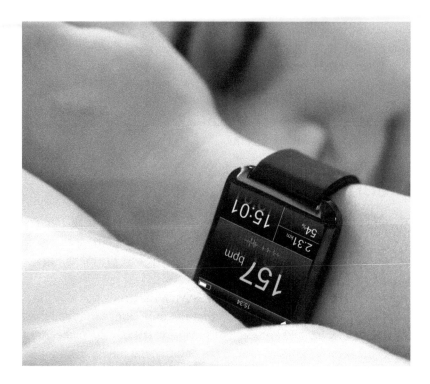

Measuring sleep

If you prioritize sleep, practice good sleep hygiene and maintain a good sleeping environment, you are 80% of the way to optimal sleep. But, I'd like to add one final piece. If you are trying to improve anything it is essential to measure the results of your actions and strategies towards that improvement. My recommendation is to measure both your success in taking action (the action being sleep), and the end goal and outcome of that action (performance). Sleep can be measured by something as simple as writing down what time you went to bed, how easily/quickly you feel it was to go to sleep, what time you woke up, how you felt when you woke up, and calculate the total hours. If you like techie-type wearables or devices, there is a current explosion of sleep tracking devices on the market. Performance is completely up to you. You will need to determine what area of your life you would like to improve performance in, and some way of tracking your progress. If your performance goals are athletic in nature, that's pretty easy to track. If your goals are improving mood, stability, communication, or anxiety—those are a little more challenging to track. My advice is to focus on a single behavioral pattern that you routinely experience (and would like to improve), and journal about how that pattern or experience is changing with improving sleep. For the executives, office workers, entrepreneurs, and employees, I recommend finding a trusted colleague that knows you well, and get him or her to consciously observe any changes in your behaviors or performance—as well as monitoring yourself. Productivity is usually pretty easy to track, as well as body composition/body weight, and eating habits. I see no limits on the variations one can try to assess their performance. It's your life. It's your health. If you are serious about improving health and performance, you will find a way to measure it.

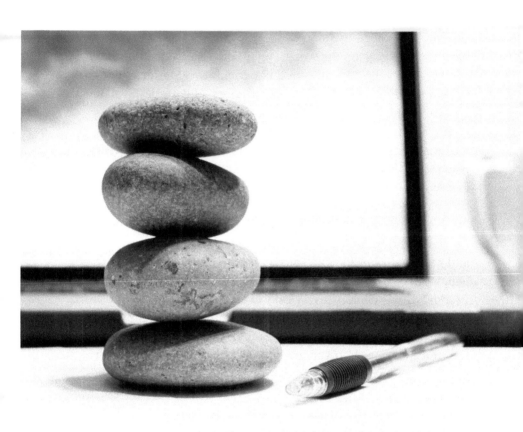

CHAPTER 9

*How to Deal With
Sub-Optimal Sleep*

How to Deal with Sub-Optimal Sleep

In this final chapter I will deal with techniques and resources for dealing with the deleterious effects of sub-optimal sleep. I will also talk about resources and techniques for getting back on track as quickly as possible.

The primary concern for most people is how to feel less sleepy during the time that they need to be awake. The obvious answer is to sleep more at night, but I also realize that might not be an option. There are several options available.

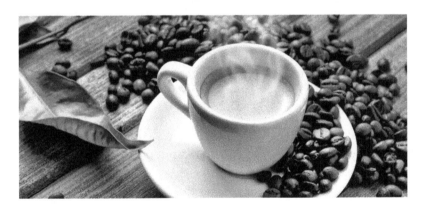

Stimulants

1. Over the counter:

    a. Caffeine is, of course the most popular and ubiquitous player. Approximately 60mg every 4-6 hours has been shown to be the most effective in prolonging attention enhancement. Approximately 200mg seems to be the most that one can benefit from at any one time— above 200mg seems to have the opposite effect for most people. I would like to point out that Starbuck's 20-ounce venti-size coffee is approximately 550mg. How quickly one clears caffeine from their system varies greatly, but, as a general rule, I recommend not consuming caffeine within 8 hours of bedtime.

b. Nicotine is also quite common. Cigarettes are, of course the most common delivery vehicle for nicotine, but it can also be delivered through dipping, chewing tobacco, mints, patches and gum. We know that cigarettes can be an extreme health hazard risk (not actually from the nicotine) and are exceptionally addictive. Addiction studies have shown inhaled nicotine to be one of the most addictive substances known. I do not believe that the same is true for non-inhaled nicotine. I have not seen any research on the topic, but in my practical observations and consulting, I have never seen anyone become addicted to nicotine mints or gum. Approximately 2mg every 4-6 hours seems to have the best effect.

c. Pseudoephedrine is available in various over-the-counter medications, and is sometimes used by people seeking to more alert and awake, or to suppress appetite. I caution against the use of this drug (or drugs in this class) as they are actually analogues of stress hormones. Routinely increasing stress hormones have a nearly endless list of health and performance risks.

2. Prescription:

    a. Amphetamines and chemical analogues are the
        most commonly prescribed. These include drugs
        like Adderall, Concerta and Ritalin. Again, these
        drugs are analogues of stress hormones, and have
        a huge potential for abuse and dependence. When
        used occasionally, they are highly effective for
        getting through an intense period of required sleep
        deprivation. However, when used chronically, they tend
        to cause habituation—meaning that you will need them
        just to have normal energy and alertness.

    b. Modafinil is a drug within its own class. It is not an
        amphetamine and seems to have much less potential
        for abuse, but has an even greater risk of habituation
        than amphetamines. I routinely hear people report
        an amazing sense of calm alertness the first time they
        take the drug, and a serial decrease of about 50%
        each consecutive day they use it. I would therefor
        recommend using it only for intensive blocks of focus
        and wakefulness.

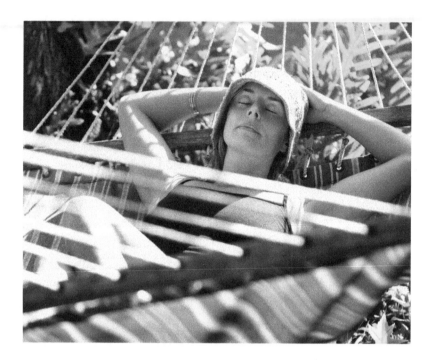

Naps

It is a common misconceptions that naps will interfere with your ability to sleep at night. Research has proven this to be false. As long as naps are taken within a few guidelines, they can enhance performance while having zero effect on nocturnal sleep.

1. A nap is defined as being between 20-120 minutes long. A 3-hour nap is sleeping, and will interfere with your ability to sleep at night.

2. A nap should be done in a slightly warm environment as opposed to the cooler environment of night-time sleep.

3. Different durations of naps have different benefits.

    a. 20-30 minutes restores alertness and creativity

b. 45-60 minute naps gives you the same benefits as the 20-30 minute nap, with the addition of improved cognition, learning, and problem-solving skills.

c. 90-120 minutes correlates with the benefits listed for the 45-60 minute nap, while conferring the additional benefit of restoring your body's and brain's tissues, and physiology—similar to the benefits of deep sleep at night.

Naps can be strategically placed during your day to enhance whatever type of performance you are trying to enhance. There is an entire book on this subject. Trying to summarize all of the information in that book would be like adding a book within a book, and I believe it would be called plagiarism. The book is entitled Take a Nap! Change Your Life, by Sara Mednick (Workman Publishing, 2006), and the correlated website is https://www.saramednick.com. This is also listed on the "resources" page at the end of the book.

Nutrition

As I have discussed throughout this book, nutrition and sleep are inextricably linked. Optimizing your nutrition will go a long way towards making your body and brain more resilient to periods of inadequate sleep, as well as increasing daytime energy and focus. Proper nutrition will also enhance exercise tolerance, which will lead to more physical resilience and self-confidence.

Talking about nutritional theory these days is akin to speaking your mind about religion of politics. There is endless contradictory "research" on the subject. So, I will leave the heavy lifting in this argument to the experts that I list on the resource page, and state my experience with my clients and my philosophy of why I believe what I do about nutrition.

First my philosophy and why: As with sleep, I believe approximating the diet that our ancestors evolved with is most likely to be the optimal diet. Natural selection dictates that those who ate the best diet would have been the most likely to procreate, protect their offspring, and survive hardship. We do know what they ate, by analyzing their bones, teeth, tools, artwork and other artifacts. It is not hard to imagine what they would have eaten by simply watching how modern-day hunter-gatherer tribes eat.

I will concede however that it is very hard to duplicate this diet and lifestyle in the modern world, and if we are going to limit ourselves to what was accessible to our ancestors, we would also need to add in the additional things that have become less appealing to us—such as eating the organs, brains, eyes and the like of animals, and limiting ourselves to animals that were not raised on a ranch.

With those caveats, my approach to nutrition is fairly simple. Eat whole foods. Do not eat things that come in a box or a bag. When you go grocery shopping, you should only be going around the periphery of the store; produce, meats, and the dairy section. Nothing else in the store was available to our ancestors, and they presumably ate the absolute best diet possible that led to this 100,000 year-old body that we continue to enjoy. Meat, fruits, vegetables, seeds, and nuts are all you need. Add some spices and additional purified fats, and you can make an endless array of tasty meals.

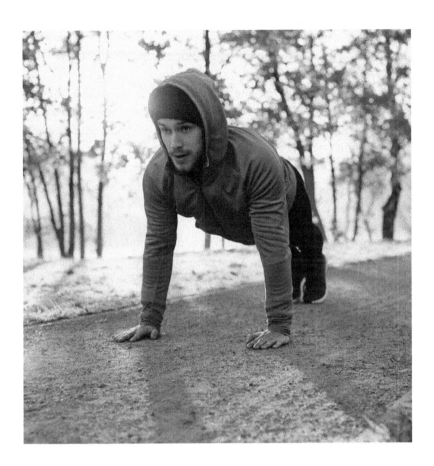

Exercise

As in earlier chapters, I will not distinguish between exercise and activity, other than to say that exercise—in my mind—connotes an intentional desire to enhance athletic performance, while activity is sufficient to maintain physical and mental health.

Exercise should be dictated by your physiologic state. If you are sleep-deprived, intense exercise is counterproductive. Do cut your sleep short in order to exercise in the wee hours of the morning. This exacerbates sleep deprivation and accelerates all of the stress hormone and their catabolic effects.

Exercising in the morning can be used to enhance alertness. The best way to do this is when the sun is well up, and you have had adequate sleep. This will fortify your circadian alignment, enhance your daily performance, elevate your mood, and make you more likely to feel sleepy at the right time of the night.

Exercise can be used to stimulate stress hormones and temporary wakefulness. Doing a little bit of exercise when you feel sleepy—and a nap isn't an option—can improve alertness more than stimulants.

If you are jet-lagged, I would recommend placing exercise in the morning if you have traveled East, and in the early evening if you have traveled West. This strategy will help you perform better in your mismatched time zone, and help you entrain to the local time more quickly.

Relaxation

Yes, I know: it seems counterintuitive right? Focusing on relaxation when you are tired. But, remember, sleep is a largely an anabolic process. Stress is a largely a catabolic process. The more catabolic our bodies and brains are, the more anabolic processes we need to compensate for the breakdown of tissues and fuels.

Stress can be manifested as anxiety, anger, hyper-vigilance, depression, moodiness, inability to concentrate, impaired decision making skills, impaired problem solving skills, lack of will power, and decreased motivation.

Meditation, breathing techniques, heart-rate variability training, progressive muscle relaxation, bio-feedback, and mindfulness training have all been shown to decrease stress hormones, decrease the physiologic effects of stress hormones on our nervous system, and cognition. Some of these have even been demonstrated to induce brainwave states similar to what is found in sleep.

Decreasing stress—through relaxation—will decrease stress hormones, and make it easier for you to fall asleep at night, and get a great night's sleep. Getting great sleep will further decrease stress hormones.

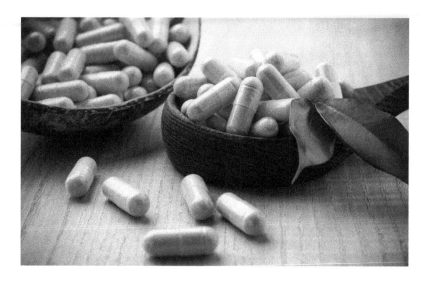

Supplements

Apart from the stimulants already discussed there are some "nutritional" supplements that can increase alertness. These are usually the plant derivatives of the stimulant (i.e. guarana is an herbal form of caffeine).

Supplements like Phosphatidyl Serine, Valarian, L-Theonine, GABA, and Kava can be used to reduce stress, anxiety, and stress hormones—while also calming the mind. Certain supplements have been proven to improve sleep. I have my own product that I developed to help the SEALs get off of sleep drugs—while I was a physician for the SEALs. You can read more about that on my website: www.docparsley.com

Other sleep supplements exist of course and are generally designed to either make one feel more calm, decrease stress hormones, or concentrate substances (in our brains) that are usually associated with sleep state. All I can say about these supplements is that I have never seen a supplement with a single ingredient be effective for many people or be effective over a significant period of time.

Drugs

Earlier in the book, I gave you my definition of sleep. One of the criteria for being "asleep" is predictable neuronal patterns. Every sleep drug (including alcohol) that I am aware of distorts these brain wave patterns. While you may get some sleep on these drugs (over-the-counter, or prescription) your sleep quality will be drastically reduced. Research has shown that people who chronically use sleep drugs (more than 6 consecutive months) have a life expectancy of 16 years less than the average person that does not use sleep drugs. It is my opinion that the drugs themselves are probably not to blame. These people are chronically sleep deprived—which is why they were taking the drugs—but the sleep drugs only gave the appearance or sensation of sleep, without the full benefits of normal, quality sleep.

However, with that said, I am not completely against sleep drugs. They are useful on a temporary basis; transcontinental travel, trauma, bereavement, divorce, legal or financial crisis, etc. If you cannot sleep at all, a few weeks or months of sleep drugs is better than nothing.

Closing

I will close by saying that this book is not even close to an exhaustive resource for sleep. My intention was to explain the basics, communicate the deleterious effects of sleep deprivation, and hopefully foster an interest in trying to improve your health and performance by enhancing your sleep quality and optimizing your sleep quantity. I believe this book is enough to get you started on your journey, but like any other performance or health tool, continued practice and improvement is where the high performers will find the highest returns.

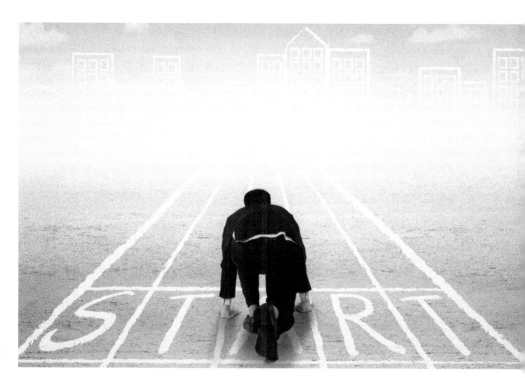

Resources

Sleep Information:

www.docparsley.com
www.thesleepdoctor.com
www.fatiguescience.com

The Promise of Sleep by Dr. William Dement
The Sleep Revolution by Arianna Huffington

Nutrition and Sleep:

www.docparsley.com
www.RobbWolf.com

The Paleo Solution by Robb Wolf
Wired to Eat by Robb Wolf
Lights Out by T.S. Wiley

Naps:

https://www.saramednick.com

Take a Nap! Change Your Life by Sara C. Mednick

Stress:

Why Zebras Don't Get Ulcers by Dr. Robert M. Sapolsky
The Willpower Instinct by Kelly McGonigal
Adrenal Fatigue by James L. Wilson

CPSIA information can be obtained
at www.ICGtesting.com
Printed in the USA
LVHW011252011219
638524LV00001B/23/P

9 781643 161341